OVERWEIGHT
IS A DISEASE

A CANADIAN DOCTOR'S
PRESCRIPTION FOR SELF-MANAGEMENT

Dr. Lori Teeple
MD CCFP(EM) FCFP

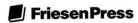 **FriesenPress**

Suite 300 – 990 Fort Street
Victoria, BC, Canada V8V 3K2
www.friesenpress.com

ISBN
978-1-4602-4864-5 (Hardcover)
978-1-4602-4865-2 (Paperback)
978-1-4602-4866-9 (eBook)

1. Self-Help, General

Distributed to the trade by The Ingram Book Company

CONTENTS

INTRODUCTION i

CHAPTER 1
MY STORY 1

CHAPTER 2
UNDERSTANDING YOUR DISEASE 5

CHAPTER 3
GETTING STARTED STAYING STARTED 15

CHAPTER 4
THE SELF-MANAGEMENT TRIANGLE 29

CHAPTER 5
SKILLS OF THE MIND: Skillpower (Part One) 33

CHAPTER 6
SKILLS OF THE MIND: Skillpower (Part Two) 43

CHAPTER 7
SKILLS OF THE MIND: Know Your Triggers 49

CHAPTER 8
SKILLS OF THE MIND: Self-Talk 62

CHAPTER 9
SKILLS OF THE MIND: Cognitive Control 70

CHAPTER 10

INFRASTRUCTURE: Creating a "Safe Zone" 79

CHAPTER 11

INFRASTRUCTURE: Eating Out 85

CHAPTER 12

INFRASTRUCTURE: Twins and the Evil Twin........................... 94

CHAPTER 13

INFRASTRUCTURE: Travel/Vacations & Celebrations................ 102

CHECK IN 108

CHAPTER 14

MOVEMENT: Exercise 111

CHAPTER 15

MOVEMENT: Moving out of Danger Zones........................... 120

CHAPTER 16

MOVEMENT: Activity & Mobility - Sedentary NO More............. 125

CHAPTER 17

EMOTIONAL EATING AND ADDICTIVE BEHAVIOUR................. 130

RECAP • REVIEW • REFLECT 141

DR. LORI TEEPLE 144

INTRODUCTION

Human beings are the ultimate survival machine. We store energy in the form of body fat as if famine were a regular occurrence. Our bodies have an amazing capacity to stash away excess food intake in our fat tissues as readily retrievable energy, not letting one calorie* go to waste. This would be great if intermittent starvation was a fact of our lives. We are set up to gain weight in a land of plenty…unless we choose otherwise.

You will learn in this book about overweight as a disease. You will also learn that the key to controlling the disease is self-management — every single day. There is no such thing as "fast and easy." There are no fads or secrets that actually work. These empty promises come and go — and often leave those with the disease of overweight worse off in the long run. Check the stats on those who lose weight quickly, and you will see that within a year they have not only regained their weight, they've added onto the original pounds. The reality is that lifelong self-management is the only way to achieve a healthier weight and a healthier you.

When people are given a cancer diagnosis that will shorten their life by years, they do almost everything that they can to get healthy and beat the odds — chemotherapy, surgery, radiation therapy, et cetera. Being overweight also shortens life by years. It is a life-limiting and enjoyment-limiting disease. Yet, we do not treat it as such within the medical system or within our culture. This book is about treating the disease of overweight using the same principles of self-management that are used in many chronic diseases.

I join you on this journey, which will involve change. Change of thinking, feeling and doing. There is no finish-line. A target weight is not the finish line. In fact, it is just the warm up. Achieving a healthy lifestyle and a healthier weight is a life-long series of choices in self-managing one of the most difficult-to-treat diseases in our culture. It is my hope that you will take the skills you learn in this book and make them your own for successful self-management.

This is not a scientific book. I want it to be accessible to all those who need the tools and skills described herein. I will oversimplify for the sake of common sense and understanding. My scientific colleagues will need to be gracious! The information I present is based in medical science and upon evidence and research, but is not meant to be technical. It is also based on my many years of experience working with patients who have made the choice to live healthy lives. Most importantly, though, it is deeply rooted in my own experience.

This is not a book to be read and set aside. Use it as a workbook to create your own guide to which you return every week to refresh your motivation, renew your skills, encourage you in your journey or to remind yourself of the importance of caring about you and your health. Go back to the chapter on eating out before and after you eat out for a year. Go back to the chapter on exercise when you find two weeks have gone by without a workout. You get the idea. Learning self-management is long and repetitive and rewarding work.

Question: What do you think and feel about the phrase "Overweight is a disease"?

_____

_____

_____

_____

_____

_____

I suggest that you pause and seriously consider your readiness to tackle your disease… for the rest of your life. Give it sober thought and read through the first two chapters. If, after that, you rate your readiness as 8/10 or more, continue on. The skills, tools and knowledge presented from chapter 3 onward will only be frustrating to you unless you have reached at least this level on the readiness-to-change scale.

*I will be using the more common word "calorie" rather than metric system measures of energy. I will also mainly use non metric terms for height/weight, etc. This simply reflects not only my demographic but how many North Americans still think in terms of these measures related to food and body size.

CHAPTER 1

MY STORY

Athletic and in-shape as a student in medical school and family medicine residency, I started an extremely busy medical practice in a rural community upon graduation…and stopped exercising. A year or two later I became pregnant. Having struggled in my teen and adult years saying "no" to food and keeping my weight down, I was ecstatic. Now I could really eat anything I wanted without guilt or shame. I stopped getting weighed at prenatal visits once I hit the 200 lbs mark with my second baby. Six months after he was born I was still at the zenith of my overweight and sorely out of shape. Thus began the next dozen years of roller coaster dieting, diet programs, fads, failures, successful weight loss and yoyo weight gain. As an emergency physician on shift work often putting in 60 hours per week, there was "no time" nor energy for consistent exercise, food planning or healthy-cooking. My children began to think drive thru fast food was a normal part of the family nutrition routine.

Then two things happened. My father was diagnosed with colon cancer, largely caused by a life of eating the wrong thing and being overweight. That was my personal wake-up call. My professional wake-up call was the second lifestyle changing event: On a Wednesday afternoon in the ER I heard the familiar sounds of an incoming ambulance siren followed by the rush of paramedics. On their gurney was a woman whose shouts and screams could be heard from the triage desk all over the department. Wisely, the triage nurse was not lulled into the trap of the "never cry wolf" response (in the ER, often those who make the most noise have the least serious condition and are treated with less seriousness). The patient was transferred into a cardiac resuscitation room — her complaint being that of chest pain. An initial cardiogram was taken, and one of our very astute nursing staff flew out of the room, grabbed my attention and said, "This woman is having an acute MI (heart attack) and she's only 38 years old." That got my attention. I quickly participated in the familiar MI routines with the staff. Part of my job was to make sure that this was the correct diagnosis. I began to rapidly ask the woman the usual cardiac questions. "Do you have a history of heart problems?" (no), "Do you smoke?" (yes), "Do you have high blood pressure?" (don't know), "Do you have abnormal cholesterol?" (don't know), and finally: "Do you get chest pain when you exercise?" She hesitated and then said, "The only exercise I get is walking around the kitchen at the burger joint where I work." My next question: "Do you eat at the burger joint?" She looked at me with one of those drawn out, eye to eye stares, and she said something that profoundly and irrevocably changed my view of healthcare. She said "It looks like I'm going to have to…change…my…lifestyle." At that moment the proverbial light bulb went on for me. As a physician I'd always known that to treat an MI successfully was very important and to revive someone who has a cardiac arrest during an MI was extremely important. In that moment I began to recognize that preventing that heart attack in the first place was priceless.

In medical school and residency, the lectures on "preventive" health were an opportunity to catch up on some much needed sleep. There was often a collective eye-rolling when the topic of health promotion was put forward. We wanted to get on to what we saw as the important stuff: saving lives and treating real diseases. However, the longer I practice medicine, the more I understand that the really important "stuff" is prevention. The 38-year-old woman with the heart attack was the beginning of a change in career focus for me. My professional wake-up call.

These two seeming unrelated events occurred within the same year. After my eye-opening experience in the ER, I began to seriously study the impact and necessity of a healthy lifestyle. It seems humorous to me now how little I knew about preventive health and healthy lifestyles back then. My study led me to realize that healthy lifestyle to manage disease was not being prescribed, or at least was not high on the list of our recommendations as doctors. There are many reasons for this, not the least of which is our defeatism based on the collective experience that those who most need to adopt a healthy lifestyle almost never get around to it…physicians and healthcare workers included. These two events were the motivation I needed to incorporate and adopt a healthy lifestyle for myself. While my habits and choices are not always perfect, my overall self-management keeps me healthy and at a more healthy weight. These self-management choices can be yours too. I share my tools and skills in this book in the hopes that others can learn lifelong self-management of their disease of overweight.

To my great surprise and relief, one of the most enlightening things I found in my research was that there is a disease basis for overweight. There was no need to feel guilty about and ashamed of my overweight condition and predisposition. The question for me, then, was this: Would I live life as a helpless pawn of genetics, brain chemistry, environment, and dysfunctional psychology, or would I take on controlling my weight and my health through healthy lifestyle choices?

This is the question you too have to ask yourself.

You will learn in this book that being overweight is a disease. You will also learn that the key to controlling the disease is self-management every single day.

What is your story?

_____

_____

_____

_____

_____

_____

_____

_____

_____

_____

_____

_____

_____

CHAPTER 2

UNDERSTANDING YOUR DISEASE

Do the math: The number of calories in one candy kiss is about 30 (or in a pat of butter or a creamer in coffee, or…sub in your own small item). This seems like nothing.

 But it's something. Starting at age ten, eating 30 calories per day MORE than you need for 120 days equals one pound of weight gain. In a year, that's three pounds. In ten years that's 30 pounds. Twenty years, 60 pounds. Thirty years, 90 pounds

People who are overweight are not gorging themselves day and night, they are not necessarily couch potatoes, and they are not weak-willed. All it takes to be 90 pounds overweight by age forty is a tiny 30 extra calories more than one needs every day.

This is a disease: make no mistake. Disease can be defined as: a disorder of structure or function…especially one that produces specific signs or symptoms…

THE UNDERLYING CAUSES OF THE DISEASE OF OVERWEIGHT (ADIPOSITY)

I am so convinced of the "disease" nature of being overweight that I have actually been using the word "adiposity" for years. Adiposity refers not to a size (i.e.: overweight or obese) but to one's tendency to put on weight, keep on weight and struggle to control weight as well as referring to the complications of overweight. Why do I think adiposity is a disease? Let me briefly (and in an admittedly oversimplified manner) outline five areas in medical study that provide credible evidence for the disease model of overweight:

- hormonal mechanisms

- genetics

- medications

- metabolism

- addiction brain chemistry

I am not suggesting for a moment that because there is a disease basis for being overweight there is no way to get it under control. In fact, what I am suggesting is that because there is a disease basis the "fix" is lifelong self-management in the same way that any other chronic disease is managed.

HORMONAL MECHANISMS

LEPTIN — A "STOP EATING" HORMONE

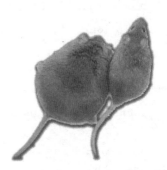

These mice are called the "Leptin Mice."

Leptin is a hormone that we (and mice) produce to control of our sense of being satiated (that is, properly fed, not too full, not leaving the table hungry). These mice are identical in every way except that the one on the left has had his leptin hormone production taken away. He does not stop eating based on being satiated (remember, this is a word that refers to having eaten adequately — not overfull, not underfed). His buddy stops eating when he is satiated because his leptin levels are normal. So the buddy leaves food in his dish when he's satisfied. The mouse with no leptin keeps eating and eating and finishes his bowl every time (and probably buddy's as well!). Over time he fattens-up while his normal leptin buddy is a normal-sized mouse.

Do those of us with adiposity have a lack of leptin? In fact, we make MORE leptin than normal people. But our brains do not read the leptin hormone signal properly. Most people with adiposity do not stop at 1 cookie, or 1 tablespoon of nuts, or 1 helping at Thanksgiving. This is not necessarily because of a lack of will power or knowledge or intelligence. Those with normal leptin control can "feel" and "know" that they are satiated. Those without it have a much more difficult time "knowing" and "feeling" when to quit eating even if it's just a few bites (remember the math — small bites count). That's part of the disease.

> *For instance: Jim bakes a pie for dinner. After having one piece for dessert, the pie goes on the counter. He does not touch it for another 24 hours; he does not even think about the pie. Jim's wife, Jane, has one piece for dessert and another few bites while clearing up the kitchen — well, almost another whole piece, not even recognizing what she is doing. Then, she thinks about the pie all evening long. Is she weak-willed? Is she uninformed? Does she not care about her health? No to all these questions. In fact she and Jim are well informed about healthy food and both have concerns for their health. But they behave in different ways about eating because Jim has normal leptin signaling. Jane does not. The causes of Jane's adiposity, while complex, no doubt include abnormal leptin controls.*

Science has not yet determined why the brain of many overweight and obese people does not respond properly to leptin hormone signals. There is a complex network of hormone and chemical control over hunger and satiety (being "full"). Leptin is just one of those controllers, but it no doubt plays a big role. Do we have a medication to fix this? Not yet. And it is my educated guess that if the leptin puzzle is solved, our bodies would use other hormonal and nerve pathways to keep us overeating, and storing fat and preparing to survive the next famine. Do not despair; there are ways of overcoming this contributor to adiposity. We will get to that in chapter 3 and onwards.

GREHLIN: A "START EATING" HORMONE

A second important hormone that controls food intake is grehlin. Grehlin is a chemical that signals the brain that it is time to eat or the body might starve. Humans probably have hundreds of internal signals that tell us to eat. Grehlin has been well studied, so I use it as an example.

Do those with adiposity make too much grehlin? Again, no. It seems that we are driven to start eating by a number of much stronger factors, while those without adiposity rely primarily on internal hormone controls such as grehlin. Grehlin is an accurate and reliable guide for <u>when</u> to eat in those without adiposity. How many times have you heard yourself or others with this disease say "I didn't eat that because I'm hungry. In fact, I don't know why I ate it." or something like that? The factors that drive a person with adiposity to eat appear to shout much more loudly than grehlin, whose soft voice as a reliable guide to eating can only be heard when these other factors are controlled — and you will learn to how to do just that later in the book.

A final example of hormone-driven abnormal eating is early pregnancy. The cravings of pregnancy make little to no sense (I wanted vegetable beef soup for breakfast, lunch and dinner…and really, I hate this kind of soup). Ask any woman who has had pregnancy cravings that are a result of the hormone state of pregnancy, and she will tell you it is not "in her head."

There are literally hundreds of neurochemical and hormonal controls for eating: starting, stopping, choosing, etc. This brief introduction to several of them should help give you a sense of the role of hormones as part of the disease of adiposity. Understanding hormonal controls assists us in developing the skills and habits for self-management that you will find in later chapters.

GENETICS

How much of adiposity in families (and entire countries) is about genetics, and how much is about our environment? This is a pretty classic nature versus nurture question. The answer is that genetics are just part of the complex equation. But it is an undervalued factor which, when understood, takes its place as one more way of viewing overweight by the disease model.

TWIN AND SIBLING STUDIES

A number of studies done in the 1990s found that identical twins raised apart and unknown to one another were as similar in size to one another as those identical twins raised together in the same environment. Identical twins as adults are far more likely to have the same body size than fraternal twins. Interestingly, siblings adopted into different families match their biological family rather than their adoptive one in terms of body size (Wadden and Stunkard's *Handbook of Obesity Treatment* — pg. 75)

Family Tree: Go to family photo albums, scan your memory and ask your older relatives, then fill in the family tree provided. Circle the family members who were/are overweight.

My Family Tree

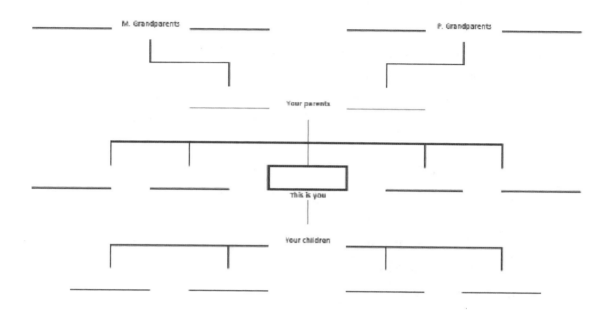

Something many people with adiposity will note in their family tree is this: There are family members from several generations ago who were overweight. This was during a time when the Great Depression and the World Wars meant that many North Americans did not have the over-abundance of food that now exists. This was also a time when many of our ancestors were very active. Many did physical work well beyond the daily labor of our generation, yet they were overweight. These circumstances in history should have kept everyone at a healthy weight (or lower) but such is not the case in many of our family trees.. There are many, many other factors at work in adiposity, but it is an interesting and provocative exercise to reflect on the significant role of genetics.

MEDICATION

Janet is a 30-year-old mother of two who has a body mass of 20 and exercises five times a week: sweat- and-shortness-of-breath inducing exercise. She started an anti-depressant for a major mood disorder. She immediately gained five lbs., and despite increasing her exercise over the next two weeks she gained three more pounds. As her physician I respected her wish to go off this drug and exchange it for another. She lost the eight pounds over the next two months without even trying.

There are a number of drugs where one of the side-effects is weight gain...insulin, anti-depressants of many kinds, beta-blockers, anti-psychotics, steroids and some anti-seizure drugs to name a few. However, it is not the individual drugs that I wish to highlight. What I would like to underscore is the fact that people who are not overweight and never have been can go on one of these drugs and begin to gain weight without changing anything else in their lifestyle. They eat the way they always did, they exercise the same way as before the medication, they sleep and work the same amount, but they gain weight. Rather than blaming certain drug classes and avoiding them (although one has to balance pros and cons), what I am illustrating is that there are potentially many chemical/hormonal/metabolic/physiologic factors that come into play in terms of weight gain over which those with adiposity may not have much control. The response some people have to some drugs has plenty to tell us about the disease nature of adiposity and helps confirm the thesis that this is a disease.

Though there are many factors over which we do not have control, there are far more factors over which we do. You will gain the skills to do so as you pursue a life based on the recommendations further on in the book.

METABOLISM

There are many known metabolic functions (or dysfunctions) at work in adiposity. I outline some of the better known metabolic-related factors to simply illustrate that adiposity is not a condition of lazy, weak-willed, over indulging individuals who live in an obesogenic nation (i.e., our nation is an environment that encourages or creates obesity). Human pathophysiology (our body systems "gone wrong") can lead to obesity all on its own despite the best of lifestyle choices. This knowledge reinforces our understanding of the disease nature of adiposity. And it reinforces the truth that only lifelong self-management can control it.

ENDOCRINE DYSFUNCTION

Hypothyroidism (low thyroid function), hypopituitarism, Cushing's disease, testicular shrinking (hypo gonadism) and other causes of low testosterone: These are a few of the more common conditions that in and of themselves cause weight gain to a greater or lesser degree.

SLEEP DISRUPTION

An illuminating study published in Japan in 2008 demonstrated that those who work night shift are far more likely to gain weight than their day-shifting counterparts. A group of 4000 day workers was compared to a group of 3000 shift workers — night shifts included. Over a 14-year period those on shift work gained significant weight compared to the day workers, especially so if they were overweight at the beginning of the study. Factors such as age and exercise were accounted for. Factors such as the amounts eaten were not taken into account because there have been a number of good studies that show no real difference in the total number of calories consumed in a 24-hour period by shift workers as compared to day workers.

Obesity 2008 Aug 16(8) pg. 1887

We know that if mice have their day/night cycle artificially disrupted, they gain weight — given exactly the same amount of daily food and exercise as their cage mates whose day/night cycles were left to nature. Interestingly, they also demonstrated very poor function in the parts of their brains that make good decisions and control emotion!

Proc Natl Acad Sci U S A. 2011 January 25; 108(4): 1657–1662.

There is a wealth of research in the area of hormone production in relationship to sleep that is beginning to explain these phenomena. Rather than studying the science, you are going to be learning how to reverse and overcome the weight gain effects of sleep disruption. As a bonus, if you are a poor sleeper you may well improve your sleep with weight loss and exercise.

Weight gain after middle-age is so common that it is almost the norm in our Baby Boomer culture. Part of the reason is the reduction in muscle mass that occurs naturally with age. As muscle mass disappears less energy is burned by the body. The energy taken in (food) that would otherwise be burned up by muscle is therefore stored in fat tissues. Women begin to lose muscle mass at about age 35 and continue to lose 7% per decade. Men start at a later age and lose it more slowly. By age 65 a woman has lost over 20% of the muscle mass she had at age 35. That is a recipe for weight gain based on personal metabolism (see below). There are ways of maintaining and even building muscle mass at middle age and beyond to overcome this metabolic factor; it just takes intentional lifestyle choices.

STRESS

The research linking stress to weight gain is well known. High stress levels bring about higher than normal levels of influential hormones (such as cortisol) that alter appetite and metabolism (energy utilization) as well as sleep.

METABOLIC "RATE"

Most of us with adiposity at one time or another have been known to say, "I must have slow metabolism." It's not strictly true. We do know that when the body is deprived of calories (energy), its metabolic rate decreases. Less energy is then burned by the body whether at rest or with activity. When the calorie level is returned to normal the metabolic rate returns to normal. During the process of weight loss metabolic rate is reduced due to lower calorie intake AND due to a loss of muscle mass, which is part of any weight-loss endeavor. This has very important implications for exercise and muscle building as a life-long self-management strategy. Those with very little muscle mass have a lower metabolic rate than those with good muscle bulk. A man with a BMI of 30 whose muscle mass is 40% of his weight will burn more energy (calories) just lying in bed than a similar man at BMI 30 whose muscle mass is only 30%.

ADDICTION BRAIN CHEMISTRY

"Food addiction" is gaining acceptance as a clinical disease by the medical community. There are some very significant findings in the brain chemistry and brain scans (PET scans) of those with obesity as compared to individuals of normal weight. The chemical and brain scan changes in response to foods/feeding in a group of obese patients in one study were almost identical to the changes found in drug addicts in response to their drug of addiction. The so-called "pleasure receptors" in the brain of an addict look extremely similar to those in someone with obesity. Many researchers think that there are also behavioral and personality similarities between those with "food addiction" and drug addiction. More on this subject awaits in chapter 17.

This is a whirlwind tour of some examples in support of the disease model of adiposity. It is by no means complete, and it is highly simplified. While these do not explain the epidemic of adiposity in our nation, they do help us shift our thinking toward treating adiposity as a disease.

I do not believe in fear mongering related to the consequences of adiposity. I believe it is only fair for people to know what awaits them sooner or later if they do not do self-management of overweight. A list of the more common disorders where overweight is a significant cause is worth reviewing:

Diabetes (90% of people with the very common type 2 form of diabetes are overweight)

Hypertension (high blood pressure)

GERD — otherwise known as "reflux"

Dyslipidemia (high cholesterol)

Heart attack

Stroke

Uterine cancer

Breast cancer

Bowel cancer

Fatty liver (in fact, the commonest reason for liver transplant in North America now is no longer alcoholic liver disease — it is fatty liver!)

Osteoarthritis

Sleep apnea

In the following chapters, I will outline some practical tools for self-management. When adopted, they will provide the confidence and skills required to get to a healthier weight… and stay there.

CHAPTER 3

GETTING STARTED STAYING STARTED

Why do you want to get to a healthier weight? Think about this seriously.

You will come back to it in later chapters:

_____

_____

_____

_____

How much importance do you place on getting to a healthier weight?

0	important	10
Not		extremely
at all		important

Compare that to:

- getting the mortgage paid off

- getting out of debt

- saving for retirement

- paying for your children's education (or your own!)

- going on your dream trip

We pay attention to the things we consider important to us until more pressing and urgent priorities come along. Our attention and efforts turn to more urgent things where there may be immediate consequences if we fail to pay attention. What happens when we fail to pay attention to healthy lifestyle and weight? The consequences are further off and much too slow to appreciate or worry about today. So we can keep putting it off year after year. Unfortunately, this disease is relentless in its course and unforgiving in its consequences. Commitment and attention to self-management of adiposity is directly related to the degree of importance placed on being at a healthier weight. This sense of importance and commitment needs to be renewed every single day, even if something more urgent comes up and presses to get in the way. In this chapter you will learn the essentials for paying attention and putting priority on your own health.

THE 7 ESSENTIALS

The essentials are drawn from data gathered from the National Weight Control Registry as well as from my many years of experience in helping patients self-manage their adiposity... and from managing my own disease. These rituals of life are absolutely necessary for a healthy lifestyle and weight. The research is pretty clear that this is what works... but it only works when each of the essentials becomes a habit.

1) ALWAYS EAT BREAKFAST

There are some excellent physiologic reasons for this. Suffice it to say that if the day does not start with good nutrition it will often end with overfeeding. For those who do not have time to sit down, even a glass of skim milk or a few tablespoons of nuts on the go will do just fine. The vast majority of successful "losers" in the Weight Control Registry eat breakfast. The Weight Control Registry is a registry of over 10,000 individuals who have had an average of over 50 pounds of weight loss and kept it off for an average of over five years and counting. While there is some controversy in the research literature around the need for breakfast it is one of the important habits of The Weight Control Registry participants.

If you do not eat breakfast currently take a moment right now — figure out how you are going to start:

What will I choose to eat:

_____

_____

What do I have to do to prepare:

_____

_____

When, where and how will I eat:

_____

_____

Now consider if this new habit is realistic for you and revise if necessary.

A great way to establish a new habit is to attach it to an old habit. For example, if you always grab your keys as you go out the door, put your breakfast with your keys the night before. Link the keys to the food. After linking for a month, you've got a new habit.

What current old habit can you attach to eating breakfast?

_____

_____

2) LOG EVERYTHING

Those who are successful losers (50 pounds or more kept off for five years or more) have something in common: They track everything they eat and drink. I compare logging (tracking) to using a speedometer. Try not looking at your speedometer next time you drive your car. I will bet you cannot stand driving more than a few blocks. The speed-ometer gives the driver awareness about speed and adjusting speed. Logging has a very similar function related to food intake. I definitely recommend an online program such as myfitnesspal.com or eaTracker or fitbit for which there are also some excellent apps. Try several and see what works for you. A notebook is better than nothing, but online programs are much better for tracking daily intake and adjusting calories. Logging programs are educational, they prevent catastrophyzing (more on this later), and they perform an excellent planning role. Go online right now and sign up (many programs are free). Begin to experiment with the program, and it will get easier. The first few weeks are a bit of work, but if I had one priority for getting to and maintaining a healthy weigh it would be LOGGING.

How am I going to log:

_____

When: _____

Where: _____

How often: _____

Do I need a "buddy" to keep me encouraged? Who can I ask:

_____

"If I do not log, I will not lose": How does that statement make you feel?

_____

If you find that last statement discouraging, do not despair. You do not need to be perfect. Just get started, and restarted and restarted as often as you forget or ignore logging. Go back to it again and again and again.

Logging is a new habit, and as I indicated above, acquiring a new habit is much easier when attached to an old one. Here are some great examples: Do you check email every day? Send yourself an email everyday with the link to your logging program embedded. Or bookmark your program on the task bar right beside your email bookmark. Do you end dinner with a cup of tea? Wrap your box of tea with a note reminding yourself to log. You get the idea.

What old habit can I use:

_____

_____

Those on the National Weight Control Registry lost their weight and continue to keep it off by restricting calories and eating a lower fat diet. You will accomplish this only if you log.

Somehow you will need to cut 300 calories of energy out of your _required_ intake EVERY DAY to lose two to three pounds per month. Logging programs will help you figure out what your required intake should be. When you build your profile the program will calculate this for you. Always rate your activity level as "low" for the purposes of calculations. For example, a six-foot-tall 200 pound man at 20-years-old requires approximately 2400 calories per day to maintain his weight when his activity level is low. If he wants to lose weight at a rate of one pound every ten days he needs to carve about 300 calories out of his diet every day. So he should log his foods and figure out how to get to and stick with 2100 calories per day. Most people — and I mean almost everyone — must carve out calories to lose weight. Do NOT count on exercise to drop pounds and for sure do NOT use the calories burned during exercise to increase your daily calorie allotment. Some of the logging programs recalculate and increase your daily calorie allotment based on the amount of exercise that you specify on the program. I advise very strongly against this. One of the main reasons I advise against this is that logging is rarely 100% accurate (even good "loggers" can underestimate their intake by up to 30%). Exercise provides you some allowance for this inaccuracy.

3) EXERCISE DAILY

SWEAT and get short of breath for at least 10 minutes at a time. That is exercise. I cannot tell you how many people sit in my exam room and when asked, "What exercise do you do, and how much per week?", they respond with "I keep active at work." If it does not cause you to sweat and have shortness of breath, it's not exercise. Activity is good, but it has never been shown to have the health benefits of exercise as it is defined above. You will absolutely need muscles to <u>sustain</u> weight loss. You will also need the energy burning effects of exercise to offset the lowering of your metabolic rate in response to lower food intake. Remember that when you cut calories your metabolism slows; you need more muscle tissue to rev-up metabolism.

For most working adults (especially those with small children), it is truly not possible to exercise daily. Get as close as you can. The ideal is 30 minutes cardio per day for five days of the week (average) and resistance training (weight lifting, calisthenics) twice a week for 20 minutes. You need not shoot for ideal right away. In fact, it is rarely sustainable to do so. Here are some ways to help you think about working exercise into your life over the next three months as you make your way toward ideal:

When can I see myself taking ten minutes to do fitness and when can I put in 20 minutes:

Monday _____

Tuesday _____

Wednesday _____

Thursday_____

Friday_____

Saturday _____

Sunday _____

What exercise will I actually do: _____

Where: _____

What do I need to do to prepare (for example, get running shoes that fit, buy an exercise

DVD, etc.) _____

_____

_____

_____

One of my own very effective fitness strategies goes something like this: I put a piece of paper on the bathroom counter where I will see it morning and evening. Every Sunday night, I list on this paper the days of the week, what exercise I plan to do that day and what days I will have "off." Here is a winter sample:

Monday — off

Tuesday — weights (calisthenics) and jog or dance 20 minutes (weather dependent)

Wednesday — jog 30 minutes or stationary bike 45 minutes

Thursday — off

Friday — jog 30 minutes or bike 45 min

Saturday — weights (calisthenics)

Sunday — jog five or seven kilometers

The best exercise is the one you will do: Dance to music or a DVD, walk vigorously outside or get a DVD for inside walking (Leslie Sanson makes some great walking videos), do a class at a gym, swim…whatever it takes. Always be trying something new. Change with the seasons. Change it up if you have a sore spot somewhere. Everyone can do something.

> *Sharon is a woman in her 50s with diabetes and adiposity, and she had not*
> *exercised much over the years. She wanted to exercise but had "very bad knees."*

She lived where there were no gyms or pools, and she worked ten-hour days. She decided one day that she had to get her diabetes under control and manage her weight. She set a goal to be able to run 5 kilometers. She started out walking in the lake near her home. One minute walk, ½ minute run (in waist deep water). Every week she advanced the running more, went into shallower water and finally began to do "walk/run" on dry land. She got to four kilometers running, and as far as I know, she's still exercising years later. She is the one who says "everyone can do something"!

Goals are highly important for sustaining an exercise regimen. What goals might be possible for you in the next month?

_____

_____

_____

In the next 3 months?

_____

_____

_____

My final word here on exercise is this: 30% of weight reduction comes from muscle loss in those who lose weight but do not exercise. That's a disaster when we consider how important muscle mass is to both health and sustaining weight loss. Ten per cent of weight reduction comes from muscle loss in those who <u>do</u> exercise. Make it your habit — whatever it takes. Go back to the questions above and review them carefully. Do not read any further until you make a commitment to start with at least one day per week of exercise.

4) EAT 90% OF YOUR INTAKE AT HOME OR PACKED UP FROM HOME

The "successful losers" of the National Weight Control Registry eat only about 10% of their calories from a restaurant or fast food outlet. One of the most important skills of self-management is establishing a food routine, leaving nothing to chance. Eating out is fraught with unknowns in terms of calories or grams of fat, salt etc. and is outside the safety of routine. Self-management means being in control. There are just too many elements that can get beyond your control when eating out. A motto that I use in my medical practice with those who must eat outside of home is *"Eat what you pack, pack what you eat."* Going shopping? Pack a snack. Lunch at work? Only eat what you pack from home. Planning ahead is absolutely key. If you do eat out, go on your logging program and figure out what you could/should order or where you should/could go. My standard "meal on the road" is a 6-inch turkey sub no cheese, no sauces — top bun removed. I know the exact calories and grams of fat. It is a safe food and allows me to stay in my "food routine." Another common alternative is stopping at a grocery store for "fast food"– ready-made veggie/fruit trays and Babybel light cheese! When I go on a road trip, the first day on the road always involves a bucket of fruits and veggies with a low fat protein packed up from home. When I reserve a hotel room it must have a fridge where I can store healthy food and avoid eating out as much as possible. Eating out leaves too much to chance, and chances are it will involve over-indulgence of the wrong kind.

5) ALWAYS MEASURE PORTIONS

There are some very elegant studies done by Dr Wansink at Cornell University (see Mindless Eating, Bantam Press, 2006) that demonstrate how poorly we estimate the amount of food/drink we consume at any one time. I do not recommend going out and buying food scales and becoming obsessive with measuring. I do recommend sizing up your dishes. For instance, buy a cereal bowl that will only hold a cup, a wine glass that only holds four oz., a dinner plate the size of your hand, and only ever use small spoons and forks. I also recommend filling your plate using a measuring cup and spoons before sitting down to eat. Serving yourself from dishes on the table means you're likely to underestimate the amount taken. You can use your hand as a good estimate for portions: the size of your palm (diameter and thickness) is four ounces (chicken and fish) and half the palm is two ounces (red meats). Your thumb is about the size of one ounce of cheese. You will learn from logging what quantity of each food is within your eating safe zone. Find a way to measure out that quantity, and use that measure forever. If you stop measuring, you will overfeed within two weeks because your eyes and mind will very quickly deceive you.

I am referring here to fruit and vegetable intake: "freggies." Five servings of freggies before 5 pm and another three before 8 pm = 5 before 5: 8 before 8. Make it your mantra. Do everything you can to get freggies into your food routine. More than eight is even better. You will be so busy and occupied with getting freggies that high sugar/fat/salt foods will fall off your radar! Cost is often felt to be a barrier. I would contend that because you will spend less on meat, unhealthy carbohydrates, treats and eating out there will be plenty left over for 5/5: 8/8. Some of us think nothing of paying 10 dollars for a bottle of wine but balk at 5 dollars for a week's worth of greens.

> *Natasha was a woman in her 40s who weighed close to 450 pounds. She was determined to follow self-management recommendations but lived on social assistance. She had about $100.00 per month to spend on food. Her dilemma was how to stretch the grocery budget to allow for 5/5: 8/8. She did it on 25$ per week! I was impressed with her ingenuity. I also recognized that her diet, though the same day by day, was much healthier than most people on a bigger grocery budget. And she lost 40 pounds over the course of eight months. I have lost track of her now but remain inspired by her determination.*

Of all the "Essentials" this one requires the most planning and creativity. Make it easier by working in batches: pack up lunches on Sunday night for the rest of the week — five buckets of freggies (five servings each). Wash and store salad greens for the week for easy grab- and-go. Make up a vegetable soup or vegetarian stew or chili on the weekend; store it in meal size containers for the week. You will come back to this when we go over "creating a safe zone of eating" in chapter 10.

What do I need to do to increase fruits and veggies in my food plan to maintain 5/5: 8/8?

What freggies do I like: _____

_____

When will I eat freggies: _____

_____

When/how will I purchase and prepare: _____

_____

7) EAT 3 MEALS AND 2 TO 3 SNACKS PER DAY

There are some excellent physiologic reasons to do this. It would seem that humans are meant to be "grazers." Our bodies function much better on a steady routine of energy intake rather than on bigger meals spaced far apart. Meals should be about 300 - 350 calories each and contain the 3 main food groups (healthy carbs like freggies/protein/fat). Snacks should be about 200 calories each and contain some protein. Men and those who do vigorous exercise (like competitive athletic training) will need to add in extra calories. Your logging program will help you figure out your calorie level. One of the skills later on in the book will utilize the concept of 3 + 3.

Choosing what to eat for 3+3 is pretty straightforward: **Healthy carbs** are fruits/veggies and very grainy whole grains (if a grain serving has less than five grams fiber it is likely not worth the calories) Stay away from carbs that are processed and those with added sugar in them. Generally the foods to avoid are those that are white or have refined sugars in them. **Proteins** are lean meats, nuts, seeds, lentils, beans, low fat dairy and eggs . **Fats** are mainly non animal oils, nuts, seeds, and meats. Stick with these, and you cannot go far wrong. You do not need to buy special foods. Modify the foods you already eat. Drop some of the culprits that contribute to your adiposity.

There is almost no room in a healthy food plan for baked goods, packaged foods, full fat dairy products, white stuff like sugar, white breads, white rice, pasta and potato fries/chips. <u>Stop reading right now.</u> Clean out your kitchen cupboards. Detoxify your space. Put these kinds of foods in the garbage right now. They are garbage. YOU are not the garbage can, so these foods do not belong in you.

The result of eating this kind of diet is almost certainly constipation unless you drink at least 4 glasses of water a day and eat all the freggies prescribed … and ensure that if you are having a whole grain carb serving it is very high in fiber.

Reflect on the 7 Essentials. These are the absolute backbone of self-management. The skills to help you achieve and stick with the 7 Essentials come next. The tools to put them into practice for life and to overcome impulsive eating, emotionally driven eating and old habits are outlined in later chapters. The upcoming skills and tools are only effective when they are used to support a life committed to the 7 Essentials. I refer to the 7 Essentials as living in a "**safe zone**." There are no gimmicks or shortcuts to a healthier weight. Even bariatric (weight loss) surgery where people lose sometimes hundreds of pounds is not an automatic pass to being healthy (most of my patients who have had bariatric surgery definitely weigh less — but they remain overweight and many are not healthier because they do not exercise and their diet is less than healthy and more than a few have regained significant weight).

Create your safe zone by figuring out how to live within the 7 Essentials. Shift your thinking and beliefs to align with these. You have a disease. It requires self-management, and these are the essentials that I recommend and prescribe. There really is no other way to get to a healthy weight and stay there. Make it your life.

PLUS: WEIGH YOURSELF EVERYDAY

How do you know when a roast is done? The meat thermometer tells you. How do you know that your vehicle needs its oil changed? The odometer tells you. How do you know when it's time to get up for work/school? The clock tells you. How do you know you have a disease that requires daily self-management? THE SCALES TELL YOU. We live by numbers in every area of our lives. Getting weighed is, however, not about the numbers. It is about a daily ritual, a daily reminder that you have a disease. Today it needs to be managed. It is not "out of sight so out of mind." Think of it as a daily recommitment to self-management of the disease of overweight. If the scale bothers you, measure your waist instead, as long as it is a daily ritual of paying attention.

I also highly recommend four glasses of water a day…it will help with the constipation that is inevitable with a lower fat diet, and it helps in the skills of delay and defer, which you will learn in chapter six.

"Today is your someday"

SELF-MANAGEMENT & SKILLS

Before you begin the chapters on "skills" some reflection on how to build skills is important. Self-management is an occupation made up of many diverse skills. Becoming a good hockey player means developing multiple skills and putting them together for success on the ice. Becoming a good self-manager requires the building of multiple skills that, put together, result in the success of a healthier weight and a healthier life. Do not be discouraged at the pace of learning new skills and becoming an expert self-manager. It is a process.

There are a number of steps in skill development that apply to the building of self-management expertise. It is very important to recognize that skills require steps some of which include failure and discouragement. Expect ups and downs in skill development. This is part of the learning process. I watched the Olympics recently and marvelled at the level of skill displayed by the athletes. These skills have been developed over many years, honed by repeated mistakes and failures, solidified by breakthroughs and personal bests. When you are learning and incorporating new skills into your daily life as part of the self-management of adiposity remember that image. The same tenacity required to excel in a sport is required for success in self-management.

STEPS IN SKILL BUILDING

Know ABOUT the skill.

You have learned *about* logging foods in chapter 3 just as I have recently learned *about* using social media. This does not mean I can use Facebook or Twitter…but I know about it.

Learn HOW to do the skill and assemble the resources to do it.

> Get started by planning what time, resources, space and equipment you need to do the skill (for instance, logging) and begin to understand how it works — read the directions

PRACTICE the skill and learn your strengths and weaknesses in easy circumstances.

EXPECT discouragements and learn from them (What if hockey star Sidney Crosby got discouraged as a kid when he could not score after a few tries?). Modify your approach because a failure or frustration is a message telling you to make changes.

KEEP ON practicing under difficult circumstances.

> As an example, the skill of measuring portions is difficult to do while on vacation. If you can practice it under those conditions then it really is a "skill."

TEACH someone else the skill.

> You will be very surprised by how much you improve your own skills. Coaching others is also a fabulous way to hold yourself accountable to your goals.

Practice with NEW SKILLS added on.

Practice really never stops for athletes doing their sport nor should it for you

doing self-management.

Practice self-management as if your life depends on it — it does.

CHAPTER 4

THE SELF-MANAGEMENT TRIANGLE

In the treatment of chronic pain and other chronic diseases, a "self-management" triangle has been developed that outlines the combination of mind, movement and modalities (things like medication/acupuncture/ice and heat, etc.) as elements of successful self-management. This triangle is easily adapted to the treatment of the chronic disease of adiposity, so it is the approach we will take. It looks like this:

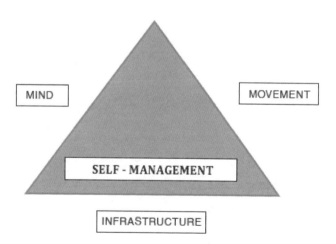

Each of the 3 parts of self-management has its own set of skills and tools. This is your disease. Adiposity is not the consequence of a few bad lifestyle choices here and there, and it cannot be "cured" by crash dieting, fads, joining a gym or going to a weight loss spa. Regaining control is a matter of making many good lifestyle choices over and over again until self-management is just an automatic way of life.

Is brushing your teeth an automatic habit? Why? Seriously, why?

_____

_____

_____

_____

The **MIND** portion of self-management is about decision making, re-training thinking, overcoming emotion-based decision making, and establishing new reflex habits and responses. In short it is about your cognitive (your thinking brain) control of lifestyle habits. It is about awareness and mindfulness.

MOVEMENT is about exercise, but it is also about activity, choosing where it is not wise to go and getting out of eating danger zones.

INFRASTRUCTURE is about the rhythm of life: the how and when and where of shopping, food preparation, travel, eating out, 5/5: 8/8, logging, etc.

Each of these three parts of self-management requires a new set of skills and tools to create new behaviors and ways of thinking for the rest of your life.

Getting Ready for Self -Management

The "when" of DECISION-MAKING:

Which is easier: staying out of a rapidly moving river or getting out of it? Imprint this image in your mind. Use it whenever you do not feel like planning ahead or sticking with the plan.

If you leave any of your eating/drinking choices up to chance, chances are your choices in the moment will be very different than those made well in advance.

When is it easier to make the right choice: making your menu selection and phoning it in to the restaurant a few hours ahead of dinner or with the menu in front of you when everyone at your table is ordering stuff you love? When is it better to decide on your portion size: before the cooking is started or when you are filling your plate? When is it better to decide your weekly menus: before grocery shopping or at the store? When is it better to decide what you're packing for lunch: the night before or in a rush in the morning?

Leave as little to chance regarding eating and drinking choices as possible. Make the plan and stick with the plan. Stay out of the river!

Safe Zone:

I live in what I call a "safe zone" of eating and exercise. Each person has to create their own safe zone that suits their life, budget, family needs, preferences, time, etc. I do not believe in giving people lists of foods or menus or exercises. Figuring out what works for you is highly individualized. I will, however, outline my "safe zone" of eating to help get you thinking. In chapter 10 you will be designing and entrenching your own safe zone.

Breakfast	2 slices high fiber, low calorie toast, 2 tbsp peanut butter, 2 tbsp. low sugar jam; coffee with milk
Morning Snack	100 -200 gm lower fat, non-sugar yogurt with 1 tsp pumpkin seeds
Lunch	6 or 7 veggies/fruit in any form — raw, cold, cooked in soup or salad form
	2 Babybel light cheese or 3 oz. fish or an avocado
	Ryvita cracker with skiff of peanut butter
Afternoon Snack	Repeat the yogurt sometimes with a left over fruit from lunch or Ryvita cracker with peanut butter skiff
Home from Work	Leftover fruit from lunch or veggies with low calorie dip
Supper	2 or 3 cups salad greens, 1 tbsp. my own oil and vinegar dressing, 2 to 4 oz. Meat (or beans or nuts) glass of wine (not always)

| Sometimes Evening Snack | Olives or 1 oz. cheese +/or 2 slices broken up Ryvita crackers |

Any food outside my safe zone requires intentional decision making using the skills discussed in the next few chapters.

WHAT IS YOUR "IDEAL" WEIGHT?

First of all, your ideal weight is the best possible lower weight for you — a healthier weight — whatever that is. Realistically only five percent of people get to their ideal BMI (less than 25) and stay there. Plan to lose 5 - 10% of your current body weight at a rate of 2 – 3 lbs per month. A drop of 10% has dramatic health benefits. For example, if you weigh 250 lbs and a healthier weight is 225 lbs, your realistic goal should be to lose 25 lbs over 12 months. Goals are extremely important. Making realistic goals is even more so. A chart in appendix one will assist you in deciding what would be a healthier weight for you. Figure out your current body mass index (BMI) then see what weight you would need to be to get to a BMI 2 or 3 or 5 points lower. Set your goal for 5 - 10% loss in body weight over 1 to 2 years. If you prefer not to live by lbs. and ounces (kgs and gms) then use a measuring tape. Get your waist closer to 88 cm (women) and 102 cm (men) unless you are Southeast Asian or North American First Nations by descent, in which case 80 cm for women and 94 cm for men is the ideal. The word "ideal" is misleading and artificial. Research has taught us that losing weight to a healthier level and staying there is what is what is important. Do not choose an unrealistic "ideal" number. Rather, choose to get to a healthier weight. The goal is not weight loss; the goal is behavior change that gets you to a healthier weight and keeps you there.

In living by self-management (adhering to the 7 Essentials and using "skill power" as outlined in the following chapters), you will achieve a healthier weight through intentional, daily planning and decision-making. More importantly, you will achieve a physical freedom to enjoy life that you may have given up on.

CHAPTER 5

SKILLS OF THE MIND: SKILLPOWER (Part One)

Look back at the "leptin mice" in chapter two and refresh your memory about normal body signals governing eating. These signals are almost completely unreliable in those with adiposity. If internal body signals are not a reliable guide then external signals must become your guide. These external signals are skills that you will put in place by deciding to do so and practicing until the habits become second nature. In my many years of experience working with this disease, I have never encountered anyone who could manage their decision-making by willpower alone. Not for more than a few short weeks! The new willpower is, in fact, **Skillpower**.

These skills are divided into two categories:

Control of <u>how much</u> energy is taken in (stopping eating): Part One of Skillpower

Control of <u>when</u> energy is taken in (starting eating): Part Two of Skillpower

"HOW MUCH" SKILLS

SKILL # 1: MEASURING — PORTION SIZING

Measuring (portion sizing) sounds childish. However, it is elementary and foundational for controlling amounts of food eaten. One of the 7 Essentials is, of course, measuring. Because measuring is a skill, more time is being spent on it here.

For the next two days do your usual food thing. Put jam on your toast, a drink in your glass, serve up your meat, make your work sandwich, grab your chips — whatever. Once you've allotted yourself the "usual," disassemble it and measure (pour that syrup off your pancake and see how many tablespoons you actually used, plus what is already stuck to the pancake…and measure the diameter of the pancake while you're at it!). Log the actual amount in your tracking program, then figure out how much of this particular food/drink you really like and can afford yourself based on calories, grams of fat, carbs and protein. I happen to really like peanut butter, so I have two tablespoons with light toast in the morning, and I have less protein and fat at supper to make up for it. You will figure out what foods are really worth it to you and those that you need to pare down to compensate. Measuring sounds like a lot of work, and it is at first. Managing any disease is work, particularly in the learning phase.

What tools do I need to assemble to measure portions: _____

_____

_____

Go get the tools and put them where you prepare and eat food.

Here is a simplified list of what you really need:

- A few tablespoons and teaspoons

- A few one cup measures

- A bowl that holds one cup

- The palm of your hand

- Your thumb

- One ounce is 30 gms (a common measure on tracking programs)

Everything other than non-starchy vegetables must be portioned. No one ever overdoses on broccoli or leaf lettuce, so don't bother measuring these. Measure out everything else.

You can use a dessert-size plate for dinner if that helps with portions, but meat, starch and grains (rice, potato, quinoa, etc.) must still be measured.

Rules of thumb are as follows:

- Use your thumb as a measure for one ounce: the thickness of the average thumb and the length from the tip to above the big knuckle. Cheese/chocolate/sausage/pate are a few examples of foods where the "rule of thumb" can be used.

- Use your palm as a measure for four ounces; the thickness of the average palm and the length/width is a great measure for fish and chicken.

- Use half the palm for two ounces as applied to red meat.

I do not give recommendations regarding which foods are "permissible" and which are not. Most of us only eat about 40 different foods in the normal course of our days. There will be those that you will eliminate (I don't eat pasta or rice, and I eat very few potatoes), but the choice is yours. There may be foods that you need to begin to eat a lot more of regularly, like fruits and veggies. There will be those that you continue to eat but at much smaller portions than in the past. I eat red meat once a week or so, but you won't ever catch me with a six-ounce steak. Two ounces is plenty (go log that in your tracking program — you will see that there is plenty of protein in two ounces and that accounts for nearly half the fats in my day).

Measuring and logging will help you decide what foods are in or out for you. It will help you decide the appropriate amounts of each food you choose. I promote a balance of foods with a lower amount of fat and essentially the elimination of bad carbs (baked goods, packaged foods, chips/chocolates, etc. — you get the idea) and processed foods.

Go back to the 7 essentials. How are you doing with 5 before 5: 8 before 8?

What can I do to get to 5/5 this week: _____

_____

_____

What about 8/8 (ie: those 3 freggies after 5 o'clock)? How can I get these in:

_____

_____

What do I need to do right now to make this happen:

_____

_____

What foods do I think I need to eliminate altogether for now:

_____

_____

Foods I need to downsize	Appropriate (new) amounts

STOP: Go back to the first page of chapter 3. How important to you is getting to a healthier weight? Important enough to measure? To do portions? To plan for the week? To figure out what works for you? **To treat your disease?**

Answer this question for yourself: If I do not self-manage my disease what will my health be like in five years based on how my health (energy, abilities, weight, medications, diagnoses, disease risk) has changed in the last five years?

_____

_____

_____

_____

In the spaces below write out "where you are at now." Come back to this chapter after a month of self-management and write out "what has changed." Put a little post it note to mark this page to remind yourself.

	Where am I at now?	One month later
Energy level		
Exercise/activity/steps		
Medications		
Sleep quality		
Sugar eaten per day (gm)		
Fat eaten per day (gm)		

Those of us with adiposity often have a poor sense of when we are full (satiety) and when we are truly hungry. Both ends of the spectrum are to be avoided. It is a skill to recognize where you are at in terms of hunger and satiety. Here is how to develop that skill.

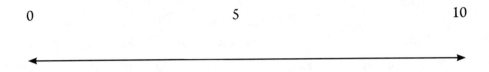

Zero

This is famished: so hungry that you are grumpy and will not only eat anything, but you will generally eat something you would NOT choose if you were at a 5. This is when seriously bad choices occur. Frustratingly, those of us with adiposity can eat our way from zero to 10 without even realizing what we are doing. It begins with being too hungry. Something in the body's "over-survival" system kicks in (one of the usual suspects is insulin levels, but there are many other mechanisms that drive this overeat reaction).

Ten

This is how one feels after a huge thanksgiving dinner when the top button on the pants has to be undone because it is uncomfortable — or heartburn and gastric reflux threatens.

Five

This is the ideal level of satiety. Find your five. Never let yourself go below a 2 for hungry. Never eat your way past a 7.

Think about where you are at right now? Compare that to feeling famished. Compare it to feeling stuffed. ___/10

Record your numbers over the next few days (put a piece of paper in your pocket or make a chart on your smart phone on which to record). This will help you get in touch with when you should eat (at a 2 or 3) and when you should stop (at a 7). Keep the picture of the scale in your mind:

Time of day	Day one Scale of 1-10	Day Two Scale of 1-10	Day Three Scale of 1-10
Waking up in the morning			
On the way to work/school			
Mid-morning			
Before lunch			
Mid afternoon			
Before dinner			
Halfway through dinner			
Mid to late evening			

Picturing the hunger and satiety scale in your mind and really knowing how you feel becomes a reliable guide for decisions relating to when and how much to eat. When you are about to eat ask yourself where you are on the scale. If you are already at a 7 you will decide not to eat yet. Part way through eating, stop and ask yourself where you are. If you are at a 7, you're finished. When you are getting hungry stop and ask yourself: Am I getting below a 2? If you are, have your next planned snack/meal right then even if that means having a "rescue" snack in your desk, your car, your gym bag, etc. The rescue snack should be about 100 – 200 calories and involve protein and non-crap carbs…i.e.: fruits and veggies, nuts/seeds or lower fat yogurt not processed sugar/salt/fat food-product.

A vital part of the hunger and satiety scale is timing. Fullness begins to be registered in the brain about 20 minutes after starting eating. In 10 minutes it is easy to eat a whole day's worth of energy, going from a 2 to a 10 on the scale before your body has even begun to sense satiety. If you eat too quickly, you can skip right by levels 5 and 7 without realizing it. This is where portions planned ahead for meals and snacks are absolutely essential. I will talk about what to do when others are serving the portions and determining the timing of eating later in the book, as well as what to do so as not to offend those who over-feed others because they speak their love with food.

SKILL #3: THE SOLUTION IS DILUTION

Energy-dense foods are a bit of an enemy for those of us with adiposity. Who wants two mouthfuls of chocolate cheesecake? There is more energy (calories/fat) in two mouthfuls of filet mignon than there is in a whole bowl of shrimp. Problem is, two mouthfuls are not satisfying. One of the reasons for this is that we have a certain muscle memory in our mouth: the tongue, the chewing and swallowing muscles have "learned" over time that many chews and swallows and even hand to mouth movements are required for our survival. Thus, it is not consciously that we feel this need to have many bites and chews and swallows. How can this be fixed? One of the best skills to overcome this learned need is to eat more foods that are calorie dilute and to eat those along with very small amounts of favorites that are more calorie dense. Satisfy the chew and swallow muscle memory without over-ingesting calories with some of these examples of calorie dilute foods:

Non-cream soups or canned tomatoes

Greens (there are dozens of kinds of greens: think outside the head lettuce), cooked or raw

Sprouts

Popcorn

Grilled vegetables (minimal oil)

Stir fry (keep the meat to 2 – 4 oz. and the oil to a minimum)

Whole grain puffed cereal

Spaghetti squash

lower fat sugar-free yogurt

Water with lemon or soda water

Low sodium V8 juice/tomato juice (just watch the labels for salt)

Put an asterix beside the food(s) that you think you can try to eat along with or instead of more calorie dense choices. For example: my supper meal plate is almost always made up of 75% salad greens (no croutons or bacon bits) and 20% meat. I don't even miss the extra meat and for sure do not miss pasta, potatoes or rice. The chew/swallow muscles have been fooled into thinking this is alright and no more food is required. Use soup to start a meal or throw your veggies and meat into broth. Try stirring wheat puffs into lower fat yogurt. Stop now and make a list of the possibilities that will work for you. Work your way through your usual eating day and imagine a dilution technique at each feeding. Commit to two of them per week. See what works and make it part of your way of life.

_____

_____

_____

_____

_____

_____

_____

A second way to dilute calories is to cut up foods into smaller parts. We're back to the chews and swallows muscle memory thing here! Do a little experiment: eat a whole grain Ryvita cracker with one hand right out of the package Count the chews and swallows as well as hand to mouth movements. Time yourself. Then take another cracker out of the package. Break it up into 12 pieces. Eat it one piece at a time counting the chews, swallows, and hand to mouth movements and time yourself again. There will be at least 25% more chews, swallows and hand to mouth movements, and it will take about 25% longer to eat the same volume of food. The muscle memory is more than satisfied, and the brain has a chance to signal you to stop.

Cutting or breaking up food into smaller pieces works very well for fruit, meat, whole grains, bread, potatoes, and low fat cheese.

In the hunger satiety scale section, I mentioned the 20 minute time frame that is required for the brain to sense that feeding has happened adequately. I have tried many suggestions over the years to slow down eating so as to get to the 20 minutes:

- putting the fork down between bites

- using a very small spoon or fork

- packing lunch components in many small, separate containers

- using multiple small separate "courses" at dinner (on separate plates)

- setting a timer for 20 minutes at dinner — no seconds or dessert until the timer goes off

- pace yourself by watching the speed of others with whom you eat

However, I've found that the most important skill is being AWARE during eating. That means not reading, working, or watching TV. Isolate eating to the act of eating. Being distracted by anything other than face to face conversation (not Skype) is a recipe for eating too much too fast due to sheer inattention. It also means making the act of eating an intentional event instead of part of some other activity. Figure out how to make your eating events intentional. Isolate eating from distractions so that you are aware of your food, your experience, and your intake. Then your mind, emotions, and physiology can register satiety. When your internal regulation system does not signal "full" appropriately, you must do so using external regulation. Make most of your eating slow, isolated events that allow your body to appreciate the fact that you've eaten well.

CHAPTER 6

SKILLS OF THE MIND: SKILLPOWER (Part Two)

"WHEN" SKILLS:

CONTROL OF EATING WHEN IT'S NOT ABOUT HUNGER AND IT ISN'T PLANNED

SKILL# 5: DELAY

By now you will be eating 3 meals and 2 or 3 snacks a day (go back to chapter 3 and read the 7 Essentials again if you are not). If we only ate what we planned for at the prescribed and planned-for times, none of us would have adiposity. The problem is that those of us with adiposity eat also when we are not hungry OR even just when we're presented with the possibility of a food or drink we love. Remember how willpower caves? Delay is a skill. Practice it. When you just feel like eating or a food is suddenly just there, DELAY for 5 minutes. This is much different than just saying "no." Delay gives you control by allowing the executive decision making part of the brain to become active. I will talk more about "executive decision making" in a later chapter. Basically this refers to conscious, intentional, rational decision-making. Set a timer, set your watch, go do something (a task, a walk, exercise) and when the time is up, decide about eating. The vast majority of the time you will have overcome the urge to eat, and you will walk away. If not, delay again. Think about where you are at on the hunger/satiety scale. If you are at a 2, eat your snack or start your meal earlier than planned. Otherwise, just keep delaying the unplanned food.

Your brain circuits can learn new timing around eating behaviors. Here is a great example: When the clock moves backwards in the autumn most of us are feeling pretty hungry for lunch at 11 am (because our body still thinks it is noon). After about a week the hungry feeling begins at noon rather than 11 am because our bodies and brains have adapted and "learned" the new eating time. Using the delay skill, you can teach your brain/body to wait before eating and put your decision making about food intake into the realm of conscious intentional choice.

SKILL #6: DEFER

Defer is similar to delay except there is an end point rather than just continual delaying. When you are presented with unplanned food or just "feel like eating" think about deferring it until the next meal or snack is due and having that food/drink at that time. Much like delay, this retrains the brain. It helps you begin to make eating decisions consciously and mindfully. Your brain cannot accept "no, just don't eat it." It can readily accept "eat it at dinner or snack time." Chances are very good that when you do eat, you will be fully in control.

Skill #7: Substitute

If you have been logging for the past week you will recognize which foods/drinks you like and will continue to have and those which are too calorie dense and have to be carved out of your eating life. Chances are, those carved-out foods include baked goods, chips, crackers, pop, chocolate and breaded foods. It may include bread, starches (pasta/rice etc.), and deep fried foods such as fries and tempura. So what is a person to do when presented with these foods or a craving for them? Substitute. Learn what foods/drinks you can use as a satisfying substitute.

Sit down right now and make a list of foods or drinks that are your usual "go-to" but you know should be your "run-from."

Here are some of mine by way of example:

Potato chips, butter tarts, pie, chocolate bars, granola cereal, peanuts mixed with chocolate chips, brownies, muffins

_____

_____

_____

_____

_____

_____

Now make a list of substitutes that you know you might like and can be reasonably successful at sustaining:

By way of substitutes, here are a few of mine:

Popcorn with no butter/coatings, puff cereal, lower fat sugar free yogurt, tiny biscotti, high fiber low fat crackers, veggies with low fat dip, flavored calorie free water, a tbsp. pumpkin seeds. A few other examples are: fruit smoothies with lower fat yogurt, skinny cow ice cream bars or sandwiches. Do your research — learn to read labels and choose lower calorie, calorie dilute, lower fat or sugar substitutes that you can have "at the ready."

_____

_____

_____

_____

_____

_____

What do you have to do to get started with these "go to" substitutes? (Remember that if it is not planned, put on the grocery list, into the cart, put away in the fridge or cupboard, or packed in the car/lunchbox/gym bag, it will not happen).

_____

_____

_____

_____

Think about <u>when</u> your "run-from" food is usually in your face. Have your substitute(s) ready.

CAUTION: HALO FOODS

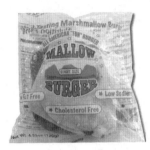

Halo foods are those "low calorie" or "low fat" healthy sounding foods. There are two things to really watch for here. One is read the label carefully. See the kids treat pictured here as a great example: the label says "low fat, cholesterol free, low sodium." Sounds great, right?

The label on the back of this little confection is a different story: 412 calories and 70 gm of sugar.

The second caution around "halo" foods is this: When you come across a food that is low in calories or "calorie dilute," there is a tendency to eat double the amount because it seems harmless. A good example is "low fat" chips. These seem way healthier than a bag of regular chips so two bags become very easy to ingest because the item has a "halo!"

When you crave, desire or are reaching for food at a time you are not due to eat, STOP. Ask yourself: **Delay? Defer? Substitute**? You have 3 alternatives from which to choose.

Pick one. Practice it. Use it.

SKILL #8: VISUALIZE

This skill is one that requires practice and a lot of mental energy expenditure, but is very worthwhile. Close your eyes and picture a food you really love but is not in your safe zone of foods (one that does not belong in your daily food plan and is no longer part of your eating repertoire). Now think about taking a bite of that food. Sense the taste in your mouth, feel the texture on your teeth and tongue, imagine the taste and feel of swallowing that mouthful. Rest for a moment and savor the whole feeling. Open your eyes.

Get up and walk away. Tell yourself how happy you feel. Smile with your face, then your chest, then your mid-abdomen. Really, I mean it. I have discovered 3 "feel happy" regions for visualizing foods. Feel the joy in all three body regions for about 10 seconds. You are reprogramming your brain. It takes practice and requires an end reward.

Practice this process 2 or 3 times.

Step 1: Find a picture of a food you love (cookbook, magazine, web page, etc.). Study it for a few seconds. Close your eyes. Think about taking a bite of that food, sense the taste in your mouth, imagine the texture and feel. Now get up and walk away. Feel happy. I mean that: Make yourself smile inside in all three regions of your body as above — feel happy. Practice this with a few different pictures. The brain should be starting to get a message and should begin to associate feeling happy with just visualizing the food rather than indulging.

Step 2: Intentionally line up at a coffee shop where there are desserts on display, a grocery store check-out line where there are treats at hand, or a corner store where many of the usual culprit foods are staring you in the face. Pick one of the foods/treats and hold it. Close your eyes, think about taking a bite of that treat, sense the taste in your mouth, feel the texture as you imagine chewing. Put it back, turn and walk away. Feel happy, smile inside and have joy in all three regions starting with the face, moving to the chest then the abdomen. Reward your brain.

This is a technique that, once perfected, will help you walk away from many temptations in a wide variety of settings including restaurants, buffets, stores and cafes.

SKILL #9: WISE PERSON

There is often an "internal battle" within those of us with adiposity. We crave and desire food (and it's never broccoli)! It sets up a battle between knowing what the right thing is for our health and wanting something very different. It is a battle of saying no to the self. We tell ourselves to delay/defer/substitute/visualize, but an argument is running in our head saying "Why not just eat it?" "It can't hurt this once." "I deserve some treat or reward." I can think of a hundred other arguments for eating what I want to eat, when I want, as much as I want and to heck with all this healthy lifestyle stuff." "I'll get back to it tomorrow," I tell myself. I learned from a wonderful social worker the "wise person" technique for decision making during this battle. It goes like this: When an internal battle begins ask yourself, "If a wise, wise person was standing next to me how would she decide?" This is giving the decision-making to the executive part of your brain, not to your disease. When the battle remains internal, the craving will win hands down almost every time. If you "externalize" the decision-making to the wise person, you will choose wisely. You will walk away. Feel the joy. Reward your brain.

More in the next few chapters about the inner battle and "self-talk."

SKILL #10: KNOWLEDGE IS POWER

Read labels and understand what the information means. Knowing what a food choice means to your body will give you the power to choose. For example, I remember on several occasions wandering around a corner store picking up a chip bag, reading the label, putting it down, wandering more, picking it up again, reading the label putting it down. After doing this two or three times, (the clerk at the counter probably thinking I was confused), I finally picked up pretzels, read the label and found it had half the calories and half the fat content. It was a better choice. Knowledge gave me the power to purchase a much better substitute (not perfect, just better). Let knowledge arm you with the power to choose. Let knowledge power trump feeling power or habit power.

Read labels always. Even if you think you are experienced in food choices. Anything that comes out of a package or bottle or can has a label. While food choices should rarely include anything processed (usually found in packages, bottles or cans), if you find yourself opening or purchasing such an item read the label. Ask yourself: How many calories? How much sugar? How much fat? Is there anything in this product that I really need (such as fiber of 5 gm per serving or protein)? If you do not know how to interpret labels I suggest the following website: healthycanadians.gc.ca/eating-nutrition find the section on "food labels" or look at www.eatrightontario-decoding the nutrition label. Both of these resources have very clear and helpful tools to get you started. Become a label expert. Know what you are getting into when you feel like getting into a bag of "run from" foods and make a better choice.

CHAPTER 7

SKILLS OF THE MIND
Know Your Triggers

There are triggers in our environment — external and internal — that signal us to react by eating. Let me give an example: Children are playing happily in the park not even thinking about ice cream. The bell of the ice cream cart rings out a few blocks away and suddenly those kids are begging for a treat. This is an external trigger. An example of an internal trigger is the deep exhaustion of working all night or being up with a sick child. At this level of fatigue, sub-conscious signals order us to eat. Thus, we must each identify our personal triggers and make a plan to counteract rather than react. The main triggers are **the five senses, stress, fatigue and emotions.** You will come back to this chapter over the coming months as you identify more and more of your triggers and figure out counteractions. Write them down, work with your solutions, and find what is effective for you.

SENSORY TRIGGERS

We have five senses. (We have more than five, actually, but these are the ones we are familiar with). All five can be sources of triggers signalling us to eat. So, let's get to work.

SIGHT

Think for a few minutes about foods (or drinks) that you simply look at and can hardly resist the reaction to eat. I know mine like I know my right hand. Chips, butter tarts, pie. I only need to see the chips at the gas station check-out and I become focused on having a bag — if not then, within the next few hours. What are your "see it and got-to-have-it" foods? Think hard — think about the places you see foods — coffee shops, check-out lines, gas stations, vending machines, your own cupboards, your fridge, the TV; this will help you identify risky situations. You can modify your schedule or avoid the situations altogether to reduce the chances that you will be visually triggered.

Furthering my example above, because I know that chips are a visual trigger AND I know that the most likely place I will see bags of them is at the gas station, I nearly always choose to pay at the pump; I rarely pay at the cashier checkout. That is my *counter-action*. Now, it is your turn to think through foods you "see-so-you-want."

Food _____

_____

_____

_____

Location _____

_____

_____

_____

Counter-action _____

_____

_____

_____

This is perhaps the most powerful of triggers. Because our sense of smell is processed in an area of the brain very closely allied with memory, there tends to be a very strong connection between smelling a familiar aroma and associating it with a memory. For example, the smell of fresh bread takes me back to being a small child in my grandmother's kitchen. A happy place, a happy feeling — and there was always fresh bread to eat. As an adult when I smell fresh bread the trigger is there to eat it — not because I like fresh white bread but because my brain is trying to recreate the good feelings of that time. I sometimes think that grocery stores and bakery places are onto this quirk of brain and memory. By wafting out great smells, folks are subconsciously led to purchase the items involved. What are your 'aroma triggers'? Think about BBQ smells, fries, apple pie baking, chocolate… Where are the danger zones in which you will encounter your trigger smells? What counter-action can you put in place?

Aroma _____

_____

_____

_____

What memory is involved _____

Location where I might smell this aroma _____

Counter-action _____

_____

_____

_____

_____

_____

_____

HEARING

This may seem like an odd "trigger," but I am convinced that certain sounds can lead to an eating reaction without our conscious decision-making. For example, when I used to hear the old hockey night in Canada music, it took me back to my childhood and the security and fun of family cheering on the Toronto Maple Leafs. Part of that scene was always chips and dip and the making of fudge during the first intermission...so you can guess what kind of food desires and behaviors flow out of hearing the music now! For yourself, think about sounds that take you "somewhere/sometime else," reminding you of good feelings and memories — what were the food behaviors or choices then? How can you counteract your impulse to mimic those food behaviours in the now when you are exposed to the sound trigger?

Sound _____

_____

Memory/feelings _____

Food behavior then _____

Counter-action now

_____

_____

_____

_____

_____

_____

TOUCH

Sometimes the attraction to a food is about touch or texture. The human mouth and tongue are covered in millions of texture sensors. Much of our food satisfaction is about texture — crispy, chewy, smooth, soft, hard, gritty, grainy, meaty, hot, cold, crunchy, et cetera. Simply the sight or thought of a certain texture can be a trigger. For instance, I am not the least bit interested in a dry, doughy blueberry muffin. But show me a moist, grainy one with a crispy top? That's a different story. Both taste the same. It is the texture that triggers the eating behavior. Do you have texture preferences? Are there substitute foods that are a healthier choice? Can you visualize that food and walk away (smiling in all 3 body zones)?

Texture _____

_____

Foods in that Category _____

_____

Possible Substitutes

_____

_____

_____

_____

_____

_____

_____

_____

Taste is the "bottom line" in most of our food choices. So how can it be a trigger? It works like this. Certain tastes signal us to keep on eating — getting more of the "taste" (and I believe texture is part of this too). Whereas you might not be triggered at all by the sight or smell of scalloped potatoes, once you begin to eat the little bit on your plate, the "taste trigger" takes over and drives you to consume more and more. Think about what foods draw you back for a second helping. Seconds are not about hunger or getting more raw cabbage vitamins into the body. Second helpings and large amounts of a food are about taste triggers. Once a taste trigger happens, the ongoing eating is really no longer about the taste. Most of the time, the trigger is flavor embedded in high fat or sugar content, both of which are delights to our brain, which keeps us mindlessly shovelling it in.

Foods I might eat too much of or take seconds based on taste trigger:

_____

_____

_____

Counter-action

_____

_____

_____

_____

_____

_____

_____

_____

Stress is a trigger in two main ways. The first is a stress hormone trigger to eat; the second is a learned behavior. The stress of not being able to make a payment, the pressure of a deadline, children who frustrate or worry us, the stress of an unhappy work place — these are common examples of stress hormone triggers. Stress, both acute (like being late for something and stuck in traffic) and chronic (like being in a no-win job situation), bring about release of extra "stress" hormones. This is a result of our natural "fight or flight" response to a stressful situation. To deal with threats (stress) in the wild, an animal must have extra "adrenaline" to fight or flee. Extra adrenaline (a neurotransmitter actually) and extra cortisol. These chemicals prepare the body to deal with the threat. The threats that we humans face today usually cannot be dealt with by fighting or fleeing in the conventional sense, but we still have the same hormone response to stress. In chronic stress, the continual presence of cortisol is a well-known promoter of weight gain.

Many of us have learned to manage stress feelings by eating; we have turned eating into our "fight or flight" activity. Write below the things you find stressful — from an empty tank of gas to a difficult teen or the illness of a partner. Write them all down. In the next 2 weeks, every time you find yourself eating in response to thinking about or dealing with any of these (or new ones), check one of the associated boxes. This will assist you in identifying your dominant stress triggers. Then you can plan ahead to counteract your "fight or flight" behavior.

_____

☐ ☐ ☐ ☐ ☐ ☐ ☐ ☐

_____

☐ ☐ ☐ ☐ ☐ ☐ ☐ ☐

_____

☐ ☐ ☐ ☐ ☐ ☐ ☐ ☐

_____

☐ ☐ ☐ ☐ ☐ ☐ ☐ ☐

_____

☐ ☐ ☐ ☐ ☐ ☐ ☐ ☐

A second major reason that many of us with adiposity eat in response to stress is that we learned it as children. The typical 'consolation' for tears in children? A treat. As adults our brains continue to make this link. The brain senses stress and a need for consolation. If consolation was found in food as a child, it will most certainly be sought in food as an adult. Think right now about what substitute you can supply for food as consolation (and I don't mean alcohol!). I tend to surf the net looking at places to which I would like to travel or looking at sewing patterns. Substituting a consolation behavior takes practice and much repetition until it becomes truly consoling and takes the place of food.

What new consolation behavior(s) can you see yourself trying?_____

_____

_____

One of the proofreaders for this book gave me a wonderful "reframing" phrase so as to pull out of the stress that leads to self-pity eating. Instead of the stress of "I have to" rephrase it to "I get to." For instance "I have to finish all this extra work" becomes "I get to finish this extra work" (and I am grateful to have a job). Or "I have to deal with these difficult kids" becomes "I get to deal with these difficult kids" (and I am grateful to have them in my life). Can you feel the difference? Next time you find yourself stressed and ready to do consolation eating ask yourself how you can rephrase your "I have to" to "I get to."

Fatigue is a trigger in 2 ways.

First, fatigue distorts good decision-making: pilots and long haul truckers have limits on hours worked because when fatigue sets in mistakes happen more easily. So too in adiposity, fatigue leads to mistakes in decision making — we step outside of our safe zone and eat our "run-from" foods. We eat more than is healthy and we just do not care because we are so tired.

Secondly, fatigue is improved by food: We have all had the experience of eating a little something that picks up our energy level when we are tired. Biologically, it really does. It becomes a problem when the food and amount are outside the "safe zone."

Can you predict your "fatigue" times? After work? Travelling? Looking after sick kids or parents?

To predict is to be prepared to counteract the food behaviors triggered by fatigue.

I know I am generally fatigued (why? when?)_____
_____
_____

so, my plan is _____
_____
_____
_____

I know I am generally fatigued (why? when?)_____
_____
_____

so, my plan is _____
_____
_____
_____

I know I am generally fatigued (why? when?)_____
_____

so, my plan is _____

Emotional triggers are different than so-called "emotional eating," which we will cover in a later chapter. The four main emotional triggers are: Happy, Sad, Angry, and Anxious.

HAPPY

In this context, happiness is being caught up with others in the moment of fun, joviality, celebration. In our culture, none of these instances happen without food (or drink). We eat because we are happy together, and we are happy together because we eat. The happy, celebratory mood acts as a trigger to eat because that's what we've always done. Without eating in these circumstances, would you really be happy? Would you be part of the fun? Subconsciously your brain is telling you "no," because eating is part of being happy and if you don't participate you will miss out. Before you realize it, you may be eating way outside your safe zone. In chapter 8, which is on "self-talk," I will give you tools to stay within your safe zone and be just as happy. Start by telling yourself relentlessly, **"It's not about the food."**

SAD

As a trigger, sadness is best described by the scene in Brigitte Jones' Diary where the main character is lonely and "sad" — she lies on the couch and eats ice cream right out of the tub. Again, as a trigger this is different than the emotional eating that arises from deeper psychological needs. The "sadness" to which I am referring here is acute, temporary and results from a well-defined incident. Food in this instance not only cheers us up from the energy boost it provides. It acts as consolation. It bridges the gap of time until we feel psychologically better, and it can help us validate our sadness in a vicious cycle. What do you do when you feel sad (or bored or lonely)? Make a list of ways to get a cheer-up energy boost, to console yourself, to bridge a time gap, to validate the sadness — none of which can include food (or alcohol). Think about behavioral substitutes:

Energy boost (eg: go for a walk) _____

Consolation (eg: chat with a friend) _____

Time Bridge (eg: surf vacation ideas on the web) _____

Validation (eg: write in a journal) _____

ANGRY

This emotional trigger to eat serves an excellent purpose. Eating is calming. It takes time, which allows cooling of emotions. It is pleasurable, which counterbalances anger, and in some perverse way eating redirects the anger onto the self where it is safer (better to overeat than punch out a co-worker). One of the tools in chapter 5 is "calorie dilute foods." Go ahead and eat if that helps when you are angry — just make sure it is calorie dilute like a bag of puffed wheat, or bowls of vegetable soup, or plain popcorn. What's your plan?

_____

_____

_____

_____

ANXIOUS

When I was growing up, if one of my siblings did not arrive home on time from driving in a snow storm my dad would often say, "I'm going to have a coffee and then I'll start to worry!" This trigger is not about chronic anxiety as in a mental health diagnosis. The trigger I am talking about is an acute worry that arises for a specific reason and causes a feeling of agitation or fear. Anxiousness is often treated with food (and alcohol). Food not only has calming and pleasure effects, it displaces anxiety for a little while from the foremost of our thoughts which, in the end, assists in finding a solution to the anxiety. For this trigger, just like with anger — eat if it suits your purposes. Just keep it in the safe zone. Eat only calorie dilute foods. Add the amount to your food log. Get on with life. In the chapter on emotional eating and addictive behavior toward the end of the book you will encounter "mindful meditation" as a means of dealing with anxiety and other emotions. You can perfect a one-minute mindful meditation in the washroom at home or work when a trigger hits. Then say no to food as the solution. Get on with life.

CHAPTER 8

SKILLS OF THE MIND: Self-Talk

"This time is your sometime"

In the last 2 chapters, you have learned about a repertoire of skills to control how much you eat at any one time and how to control getting started in the first place.

How are you doing with portion sizes? What do you need to do to get with it?

_____

_____

_____

How are you doing with the "hunger and satiety" scale? Ask yourself — "am I eating beyond a 7/10? At what meals, snacks? What kinds of occasions? What kinds of foods?" Once you've figured this out — you can fix it:

_____

_____

_____

How are you doing with substitutions? What is working? What else can you try this week based on the "run-from" food you are having trouble with?

_____

_____

_____

_____

If you are not logging — you are not losing or controlling weight. Bottom line.

This chapter is a collection of "self-talk" phrases. In the treatment of addictions such as smoking or alcohol, self-talk is an important component of changing brain interconnections and nerve wiring so as to change behavior and eventually make that behavior almost automatic. For many of us with adiposity, there is an element of addiction; it is a behavioral addiction with some chemical involvement as well (more on this in chapter 17).

Self-talk is a skill and is used along with the skills in Chapters 5 and 6. Make these phrases your own:

"HUNGER IS FAT TISSUE (ADIPOSE) LEAVING THE BODY"

This is analogous to the army phrase, "Pain is weakness leaving the body." There will be times with self-management that you feel hungry. I **only** recommend feeling hungry at bedtime, but if it happens unexpectedly and you begin to have that withdrawal feeling (desperate to eat) but the only food around is a "run-from," tell yourself "hunger is adipose tissue (fat) leaving the body." Revere the moment. Do not be frustrated, anxious or angry. Think of how good it will feel to have a snack/meal when the time comes and how good it feels to stay in control. Go with it.

"IT'S NOT ABOUT THE FOOD"

I once worked with a patient who was doing self-management beautifully. She was aiming for a trip to California, and her goal was to sustain her 40 lbs weight loss while on vacation. When she returned and had in fact lost a few pounds I asked her, "How did you do it?" She is the one who said, "It's not about the food." The enjoyment of the good time was not about the food.

How many times do we go out for lunch, on a vacation, to a party or family gathering and reach for the food as if it was the source of the "good time?" Or mindlessly eat because food is part of celebration habits in almost every culture? We will talk more about this in the chapter on twins.

Describe a time recently when you were fooled into thinking "It's about the food," and reflect on how you would do it differently:

_____

_____

_____

_____

Next time you are going into a circumstance where it is usually "about the food," practice this self-talk. Prepare yourself — think of substitutes, visualize, delay, measure portions, take a small plate — choose one of these to help maintain the mindset that "it's not about the food."

"IT MATTERS NOW"

The next bite MATTERS, and it matters NOW. Not tonight, not tomorrow or next week. When your health is on the line, it matters now. If you had pneumonia, you would never dream of putting off your antibiotics to maybe tomorrow or next week. I've never heard a cancer patient say, "Maybe I'll just put off that chemo and give my disease a little longer to do me more harm." Because the consequences of adiposity are not immediate and the consequences of "this bite now" seem insignificant, this self-talk phrase is extremely important. "It matters now" is particularly important after being out of control with eating for a snack, a meal, or longer. Decide NOW. When you miss a dose of antibiotics, the next dose is even more important. Apply this mindset to "it matters now."

Picture yourself in a typical circumstance in the recent past where you have said to yourself "this time it doesn't matter — I'll be 'good' next time." Do a long, slow inventory of that circumstance (what led up to it, where you were, who or what triggered you, what were you thinking etc.):

_____

_____

_____

_____

_____

Now apply an "it matters now" phrase to the circumstance you've written about.

What would you have done differently? Because that is what you will do next time!

_____

_____

_____

_____

_____

"WILL THIS FOOD DELIVER WHAT IT PROMISES?"

If you ever pause to gaze at a food you love and have that inner struggle — wanting it but knowing better — STOP and ask yourself: "What is it I feel this food will deliver?" "What is it promising me?"

_____

_____

_____

_____

_____

HAS FOOD EVER DELIVERED ON THIS PROMISE FOR YOU? How did you feel the last time you chose the empty promise?

_____

_____

_____

"DON'T CATASTROPHIZE"

Often, if you get out of your "safe zone" for a meal, a day, or a week and feel as if you have "blown it" in terms of self-management and control of eating, the automatic impulse is to say, "I've blown it now, might as well give up. I can't do this lifelong, day-in-day-out lifestyle, I've never been any good at this kind of routine, all my hard work is ruined, I knew in my heart I would be a failure...." Any of those phrases sound familiar? These kinds of sentiments are called "catastrophizing." One of the benefits of catastrophizing is that we are letting ourselves off the hook. It looks like we're discouraged and giving up and resigned to our failure because it is just too hard. Not so. Catastrophizing is our way of avoiding the next good self-management decision. There is no such thing as a catastrophe. There is no such thing as failure. It is only a catastrophe if you never get to starting over, and over, and over, and over. Make the next good decision and move on. An excellent way to prevent catastrophizing is to log in the food(s) that you believe you have "blown it" by eating. Almost always you will see it is not as bad as you thought when you were busy berating yourself! Give yourself permission to NOT be perfect.

When was the last time you heard yourself "catastrophizing?" What were the circumstances and what did it take to get back to daily self-management?

_____

_____

_____

_____

_____

_____

DR. LORI TEEPLE

"CRAVE BUT DON'T CAVE"

Craving a food or drink is not a sin, and it doesn't mean you have to lose control of decision making. Craving is a physiologic thing. That is, it is rooted in neuro-hormonal mechanisms. Anyone who has been pregnant can verify that craving is beyond just "thinking" or "feeling" about a food. I recall being pregnant with my first child and longing (in fact, begging) for vegetable beef soup — breakfast, lunch and dinner as I illustrated in chapter two. I did not even like this kind of soup, but something was driving me to search it out beyond all reason. I believe that we all crave certain foods/drinks — it is inevitable. However, we do not have to "cave." Acknowledge the craving, accept it, understand it and prepare for it. Here is a great example: If you love butter tarts and the minute you encounter one you begin to crave it, a small voice of unreason in your head gets louder and louder. Stand up to that small voice. Accept the craving, tell yourself the truth and choose not to cave. Be prepared — you know where this food will be (think bakeries, coffee shops, check outs), so either avoid the location or have a plan of encounter.

"IT'S NOT TOO LATE"

If you ever choose a food (put it on your plate, order it, pick it up at a café or store) and suddenly have a second thought like, "I know this is not in my safe zone," listen to that voice. It is NOT TOO LATE! Take that item to the nearest garbage — ditch 75% of it and walk away. Smile with your face, then your chest, then your abdomen. Every time you make a choice like this you reinforce and strengthen good decision making that keeps you in your safe zone.

"3 GOOD THINGS THAT WILL HAPPEN WHEN I WALK AWAY"

When faced with a "run-from" food, no matter where you are chances are it is too hard to "just say no." Instead, I recommend listing three good things that will happen to you when you do not indulge. My three things are: 1) I will feel very happy when I've walked away, 2) My clothes will fit me better when I've walked away, and 3) When I walk away this time it makes me more powerful for next time. Now, you decide on your own 3 good things:

1) _____

2) _____

3) _____

"I GIVE UP" VERSUS "I JUST CAN'T DO THIS TODAY"

Can you feel the difference? So often in the self-management of adiposity, the road is too hard. We flag and fail and we make wrong turns. Sometimes you will be so far from the 7 essentials that you just feel like giving up. Turn that sense of giving up for good into TODAY only. Tomorrow is a new start…always.

"FAILURE IS JUST A CHANCE TO LEARN"

In fact, sometimes I tell patients that I want them to have a setback in their self-management so that we can troubleshoot it and learn something that will help in the future. Write down the "failure", and write out all the steps that led to it. Then write down how you will interrupt that sequence of events or factors in the future. Here is an example: I just ate a big brownie. This so-called failure actually started with wanting coffee but having no cash. I went into a café knowing there were treats there and knowing that I would have to buy a few things to warrant using my debit card, thus rationalizing the brownie. Analysis: go to the ATM first. Pay cash for the coffee. Visualize the brownie. Walk away. Smile.

Reflect on your last "failure." What did you learn?

_____

_____

_____

_____

_____

_____

Procrastination is a form of lying to the self. Lying is about denying an unwanted reality. The reality is that continuing with my current behavior is killing me. Slowly. My current behavior is robbing me of energy and vitality and enjoyment of life by limiting my physical and mental abilities. If I do not change my behavior starting today, starting now (or restarting now) I will not be able to do the things I want to do in the future. The consequences of my disease are only going to get worse. These are reality statements. Procrastination is a powerful lie we tell ourselves. Challenge the lie. This time is my sometime — today is my someday. Use this self-talk statement every day. Use it when you get on the scales, use it when you pack your food for eating outside the house, use it when you walk away from a "run-from" food and smile, use it when you are out with friends, use it when you pass the drive-thru.

"IT'S NOT ABOUT LOSING WEIGHT — IT'S ABOUT BEHAVIOR CHANGE"

Changing behaviors one after another, skill by skill, situation by situation, day by day is the goal. Getting to a healthier weight will follow. Maintaining a healthy weight will be achieved. Reward behaviour rather than weight loss. Reward good choices. Set goals about behaviour. For example, every time I exercised on a recent conference trip away from home I put a check mark on my exercise list. I achieved 6 out of 7 on my list so when I got home I rewarded myself (and I am still enjoying that new bike shirt). Make a list of rewards that work for you. Reward the behaviors. The healthier you, the healthier weight will automatically follow the behaviors.

CHAPTER 9

SKILLS OF THE MIND: COGNITIVE CONTROL

So far you have done a lot of work with skills and tools for getting to a healthier weight. You have the 7 Essentials down, and you are weighing yourself daily. If this is not true, go back and start over again. Do not keep going in the book hoping somehow you will "catch on." There is nothing easy or quick-fix in self-management. You will find your "aha" moment way back in chapter 2 or 3. Stay there until you do. Self-management of adiposity is about changing the mind and behaviors, building the infrastructure to support a healthy weight and getting to the movements that sustain weight loss.

In this last chapter of the section on "skills of the mind," the focus is on cognitive or executive decision making. When you achieve executive control over food and exercise decisions, you are fully in charge of your healthy weight self-management. Some definitions are in order. Executive decision making refers to the "thinking," to the in-charge part of the brain. In medicine, we often refer to the frontal lobe (or more accurately the prefrontal lobe) as the executive branch of the brain. We need the prefrontal lobe to make good decisions in all parts of our life, to keep us well behaved socially, to screen out our destructive impulses, to analyze, synthesize and interpret information and allow us to act on it in intelligent, mindful, and thoughtful ways.

By way of contrast, when a person sustains damage to their prefrontal cortex or has it removed, they often become inappropriate. They might undress in public, shout at anyone at any time, curse and swear, urinate on the floor, act out sexually with little to no impulse control, eat non-stop, et cetera. These folks have lost their executive decision maker. With respect to food, sometimes those of us with adiposity function like we too have lost our executive decision maker. The prefrontal area of the brain is missing in action.

Humans can ignore their prefrontal cortex very well. We call this denial. Denial is one of the most powerful mechanisms humans possess to protect them from an unwanted reality. I want to address the power of the brain in this self-deception because in the disease of adiposity there is a high degree of denial around the health consequences of aberrant (abnormal) food behavior. This is what allows us to continue with the behavior in spite of how it damages us. Denial is highly powerful. I learned this lesson one day early in my career as an emergency physician.

> *It was a Saturday morning emergency room shift. A young woman showed up at the triage desk with abdominal pain. The nurse took her vitals and her medical story specifically asking her about symptoms, her last period and the possibility that she could be pregnant. The young woman denied any possibility of pregnancy and said she was having regular periods. From triage she was transferred to an examination room where another nurse took further history and did a preliminary exam. Again, she denied the possibility of pregnancy. The nurse came out of the room and said to me, "She's pregnant — I'll bet my license on it." It was my turn to interview this young university student who again denied any possibility of pregnancy and was certain she had regular periods. I examined her — and broke the news to her that I could feel a baby's head when I did her vaginal exam. She was stunned, but not as stunned as I was when she asked me if I could call her husband! The shocking thing about this story was the husband's incredulity (he refused to believe me on the phone). Two hours later they had an 8 lbs baby boy. These were two intelligent university students both in denial for nine months about a reality otherwise impossible to ignore.*

Denial around adiposity is even more powerful. The capacity of the human brain to sustain behaviors of self-destruction while feeling good about it speaks to the power of brain wiring gone wrong.

So, how do you get your "prefrontal lobe" working for you? How do you get to cognitive control of eating and exercise? How do you harness executive decision making? You will do so by strengthening the brain pathways of cognitive control, developing and using these nerve pathways to such an extent that the pathways of aberrant (wrong choice) eating become nearly extinct.

I am going to walk you through a very simplistic model of the brain and 4 main pathways that can be altered to gain cognitive control:

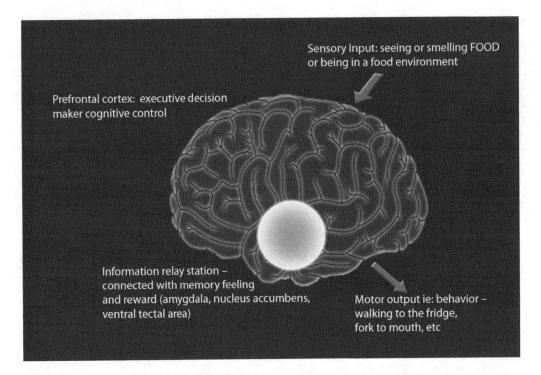

The ordinary way these pathways or circuits work is as follows: Sensory input (like seeing a bag of chips) signals the information relay station, then a FAST signal goes to the motor output section, and voila — food behavior (the straight arrow lines represent a fast bypass freeway). One might well refer to this as a reflex. By contrast, SLOW signals (represented by the curving lines in the second picture) are sent from the information relay station to the prefrontal cortex, then back to the information relay station and then on to the motor output pathway. But, alas, this happens too slowly for executive or cognitive (prefrontal) control of food decision making or behavior change in response to sensory input.

DR. LORI TEEPLE

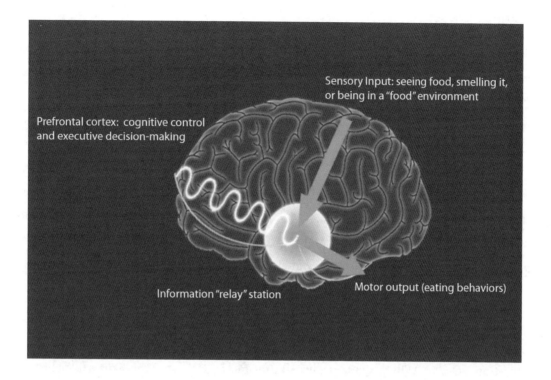

One of the reasons sensory input signals follow the "fast" bypass route to the motor output (behavior) section of the brain is that we use this pathway so often that it has become the "freeway" for the signals that control eating. The signals to the prefrontal cortex move along slowly because this pathway is rarely travelled and is in disrepair (not quite, but you get the idea). The pathway back to the information relay station from the prefrontal cortex (gentle curved line) is also a slow one so that signals from the prefrontal cortex that could govern food behavior are too little, too late to influence the information relay station and thus behavior.

How can the pathways be changed? How do we teach our old brain new tricks? How do we extinguish some of the reflex (bypass) pathways and strengthen the slow ones that work in our favor for managing adiposity?

LIMIT SENSORY INPUT

Remember your triggers? In the chapter on knowing your triggers you have already learned about avoidance of certain foods or situations. This is part of limiting sensory input. Go back to that chapter and review your sensory triggers. Review your "counteractions"; what is working for you?

The skills of delay and defer allow time for the "slow" pathways to conduct signals to the prefrontal cortex. The sensory signal enters the brain and heads for the information relay station where "eating as a reflex" will happen **unless** you can redirect the signal to the prefrontal cortex. Delay and defer are two ways of redirecting. The more often these skills are used, the more dominant the pathway to the prefrontal cortex becomes (and the weaker the pathways for reflex eating become). As the pathway to the prefrontal cortex gets stronger and speedier, more and more food signals will be processed there rather than bypassing. When the prefrontal cortex is given a chance it will send good decision making signals to "motor output" resulting in controlled eating behaviors. While it may seem tedious to set the timer or your watch so as to delay, think of it as brain retraining, cognitive reshaping and putting your prefrontal lobe to work for you.

QUESTION SENSORY INFORMATION

Questions such as "Will this food really make me feel better?" stop the signals from hitting the bypass pathway immediately. Questions force sensory signals to go to the prefrontal cortex for processing (analysis, synthesis, interpretation, et cetera) so that a good eating decision can be made and acted upon. Learn to question everything outside your safe zone. Refer back to earlier chapters for a list of great questions about food sensory input:

Where am I at on the hunger/satiety scale?

What would a wise person tell me to do in this circumstance?

Did eating like this deliver on its promise in the past?

Is it (fun/happiness/feeling good) really about the food?

Why does it matter "now?"

Does craving have to mean caving?

Is there a substitute for this food?

Continue this list on your own:

_____

_____

_____

_____

The more you question yourself, the more sensory input signals are diverted to the prefrontal cortex, and the pathway becomes stronger. Have a few standard questions at the ready for yourself because sensory input is happening all the time — when you are in your own space and when you're out, when you read a menu or a magazine, when you see TV or advertisements, when celebrating with friends or going to the grocery store, on and on and on. Find the questions that give you "sober second thought" — this is what allows sensory signals to be diverted to the prefrontal cortex and good decisions are made about eating behaviors and choices.

GIVE YOUR PREFRONTAL CORTEX SOME EDUCATION

In order for the prefrontal cortex to analyse and interpret sensory signals such that good decisions are made about food and exercise behaviors, the brain needs correct information with which to make good decisions. If you have no idea that deep fried chicken is not healthy for you, the prefrontal cortex will not stop you from eating it. In creating your "safe zone" of eating, you are giving your brain a great education. Knowledge really is power in this circumstance. Reading labels is fabulous education, and logging contributes to your knowledge base in significant ways. Later in the book I will give you information on exercise that your prefrontal lobe can work with. Read about food and food behaviors from reputable sources (Dietitians of Canada, Heart and Stroke Foundation, American Heart Association, Mayo Clinic). One of my greatest skills in the convenience or grocery store is to read the labels of the food in my hand, giving information to my prefrontal lobe and creating an opportunity to be guided away from poor choices.

GIVE YOUR PREFRONTAL LOBE "PRE-PACKAGED" THOUGHTS

In the last chapter, one of the "self-talk" skills was to list 3 good things that will happen if you walk away. This is a good example of pre-packaged thoughts. Whether we are aware of it or not, how and what we <u>think</u> in advance of a situation significantly determines our behavior. Thinking pre-packaged thoughts will activate the prefrontal cortex before sensory input has a chance to set reflex pathways in motion. As you walk into a restaurant, use your pre-packaged thoughts. As you start a family dinner or BBQ, use your pre-packaged thoughts. You get the idea. What is your next "event?"

_____

_____

_____

_____

What pre-packaged thoughts are you going to use?

_____

_____

_____

_____

REWARD GOOD CHOICES

I really cannot say this enough. The "fast pathways" have an amazing built in reward system. Food has its own reward (pleasure) centers in the information relay station area of the brain very similar to the reward centers for addictive drugs such as cocaine and narcotics. High fat and sugary foods in particular signal the pleasure centers, which makes us feel rewarded. Thus when we deny ourselves the foods of our craving, it seems to these parts of our brain that we are punishing ourselves. This is why it is so vital that you learn to reward each and every good choice. Doing so strengthens the slow pathway from the prefrontal cortex back to the information relay station, and good behaviors result. Rewards are not for actual pounds lost — rewards are a means of consciously reinforcing good choices that will lead to weight management. The more these choices are reinforced through reward, the easier it becomes to make good choices. The prefrontal cortex more readily sends good choice signals to the information relay station, which then signals our motor output station to carry out good choice behaviors.

Rewards ought to be in two forms: ultra short term and short term. An ultra short term reward would be something like putting a bead or a one dollar coin into a little bucket in the car everytime you go into a Starbucks and visualize a treat but come out with only the coffee. Another ultra short reward is putting a simple check mark or star on the calendar for every day that you exercise (actually, in our medical practice we have a magnet board for staff — every time any one of us exercises on any given day we get to put a magnet behind our name. Silly but effective). The reasoning behind ultra short term rewards is this: Otherwise good choices can feel like punishment, and brain pathways will not respond to punishment and deprivation. Shame and guilt are reverse motivators in my experience.

Figure out what ultra short term rewards might work for you (stars on a calendar, beads in a glass dish, coins in a jar, etc.):

_____

_____

_____

_____

Short term rewards for good choices stimulate the brain's motivation circuits which are critical for developing new behaviors. Let's say that the prefrontal cortex receives a signal from sensory input about the number of calories or fat content on a food label. The executive decision maker analyzes this information and sends direction to the information relay station to dictate the behavior of putting the food back on the shelf. This requires a lot of motivation — brain energy, actually. It would be much easier for the brain to default back to bypass pathways. Rewards provide motivation energy.

When I am on my own, away from home in a city across the country, it would be very easy to eat whatever, whenever because, as we will discuss later, it is hard work to stay in the safe zone on the road. I always set myself a short term reward to keep my executive decision pathways on their game. If I stick to my regimen (at least 90%) then I get to have the reward. This can be anything from a pair of biking socks to junk jewellry to something really nice like a manicure. The same goes for exercise — sticking to the game plan requires a reward system.

Short term rewards are for good choices over a longer period of time — like a week or a few weeks at most. A month is too far in the distance. If your ultimate reward is a trip six or twelve months from now it is too vague to be a motivator. If you set aside cash for a trip on a weekly basis as a reward for executive choices and put the pile of cash where you can see it everyday, then you have a short term reward system for motivation.

Make a list of potential short term rewards for sustaining motivation and the time interval that will work for you.

CHAPTER 10

INFRASTRUCTURE
Creating a "Safe Zone"

CREATING A "SAFE ZONE"

People with a chronic disease learn to live in a way that keeps them as healthy, active and safe as possible. For example, someone with advanced Parkinson's disease lives in a "safe zone" that includes getting a full night's sleep, resting during the day, taking medications on a tight and rigid schedule, keeping their living space clear of obstacles to walking, using grab bars in the bathroom, and employing a walker for mobility. Those of us with adiposity have a chronic disease. So what are the "safe zone" elements required to manage this disease? Many of these elements look like the 7 Essentials, so you are already halfway there to creating your safe zone if you are living by the essentials (and weighing yourself daily).

AN EATING SCHEDULE

To successfully manage the chronic disease of adiposity, routines are absolutely essential. If eating is left up to chance the most likely outcome is that overeating and eating the "wrong" thing will be the result. Find a way to eat 3 meals and 2 to 3 snacks a day; set up your regimen and stick with it no matter what you are doing or where you are. How are you doing with this? What needs to change? How will you make this change? Stop: *Figure it out right now*. Remember that creating a new habit will be much easier if it is "stuck" alongside an old one.

_____

_____

_____

_____

_____

_____

A FOOD ROUTINE

In chapter four there is a short reference to a "safe zone" in which I listed my own food routine. Now that you have been logging and using skills of the mind and doing self-talk for a few weeks or months it is time for you to formalize your own food routine. This is a list of foods (and drinks) that you will have at each meal and snack 90% of the time. Use foods you actually like — modify them to fit your calorie/fat/protein requirements if needed (if you are logging on a program you should have a very good handle on this by now; if you don't then stay with me, you will get there). For SURE the portion size has to be part of this routine (do not write "steak" — write 2 oz steak, i.e.: half the size of your palm). For SURE the words "low fat" or "sugar free" should be part of this routine as well. And for SURE, for SURE, the routine has to include 5/5: 8/8.

_Breakfast:_____

_____

First snack: _____

_or_ _____

Lunch: _____

_____

Second snack (time? Place?) _____

or _____

*Supper:*_____

_____

Evening snack (if required) _____

or _____

There is a certain boredom to this rhythm of foods — but boredom is safety. Is it boring to take the same old heart pills three times a day, day after day? For sure, but the routine is part of managing heart disease. Overweight is a disease. Routines are an essential part of self-management. Once you have an established safe food routine, you can begin to exchange foods for new but equivalent ones. Replace lettuce with spinach — see if you like that. Replace low fat cheese with tuna as a protein — see if that works for you. You get the idea. Establish the food routine FIRST — entrench it. Follow it the way you follow your routines of getting out of bed and dressing.

GROCERIES

Always have a list. Always have a list — did I say that twice?! Shop at the same place and in the same fashion as a habit. Start in the fruit and veggie section and then go around to the (low fat) dairy and meats. Skip the bakery aisle. Skip the aisles with processed foods. Skip the aisles with junk foods (limit that sensory input!). Find out where the cereal or bread that YOU have in your food routine is stocked — go straight there. Get in and get out. Do the same with beans or other canned goods. Shop like a robot — make none of your own decisions on the spot. Get ready to visualize the treats at the check-out and prepare to smile at yourself as you walk away with your grocery cart. If all of this is just too overwhelming, send someone to shop for you with a very specific list.

Another very helpful tool is to manage the size of your grocery cart. Do this little experiment a few times to help yourself develop a new and healthier shopping system: Bring two bungee cords with you to the store. Clip them in an X pattern about two-thirds of the way down the length of the cart. That big first two-thirds is for fruits and veggies and low fat dairy. The last third of the cart is for meats, whole grains, etc.

PREPARATION SCHEDULE

What preparation schedule do you need to keep so that getting your 5/5: 8/8 will happen? I need to make a vegetable soup or veggie chili of some sort every Sunday so as to have readily available lunch material. I also need to prep all my raw vegetables and fruits for the entire week and separate them out into plastic containers to grab for lunches or car trips or meetings. I do this task on Sunday evening and the soup thing in the afternoon. Groceries are usually done Sunday at noon. Sunday night dinner includes salad so all the salad greens are washed and ready in plastic containers in the fridge for dinners and the salad dressing for the week gets made at the same time. One of the keys to sustaining a food routine and eating schedule is to have the foods easily available and ready when you need them. You can save a lot of time and energy by doing all food preparation tasks at one time. You need only motivate yourself to do this once a week. I make it a rewarding experience by listening to music I love and having a glass of wine when everything is done. Design a preparation schedule that works for you.

Veggies: _____

Fruit: _____

Salad greens: _____

Veggie soup/chili/etc.: _____

"To go" foods (lunches, etc.): _____

Before every flight, a pilot goes through a routine check list to ensure that the plane and the staff are fully prepared and that everything is in excellent working order. Every flight, every time — the routine of preparing for all eventualities and staying safe. Your routines of preparation for eating serve the very same function. Is it a chore for the pilot to do the same routine again and again? Is it absolutely essential?

EAT WHAT YOU PACK / PACK WHAT YOU EAT

Those of us who eat a meal or snacks at work or on the road need to live by this motto almost daily. In my clinic, there are foods outside my safe zone lying around in the kitchen most of the time. Very kind folks who wish to express their gratitude to our staff make home-made "goodies" (actually, they are generally "baddies"). Our staff lunch table is absolutely covered with boxes of nuts and chocolates at Christmas. Eat (only) what you pack; pack what you eat. In my workplace, I must stay out of the lunch room at Christmas, ask staff to hide the baddies, openly brag to my colleagues that I won't be having any of 'this' food (this is a great trick of accountability). Think about what you need to do in your lunch/snack places to limit sensory input and stay in your food routine. Pack what you are supposed to eat, and eat that only. Leave nothing to chance.

CHOOSE ONE SAFE FAST FOOD ITEM AND STICK WITH IT

We will cover more of this in a later chapter. For now I suggest that you start some research about what "fast food" on the road is safe for you and fits within your food routine. Mine is a 6 inch turkey sub — no cheese, veggie toppings only, no sauces. Go to the website of common fast or slow food places, and go over the labels looking firstly at the serving sizes (often a serving size is ½ a burger — but the whole burger is what we eat!). Then look at calorie and fat content. Find a food you like that fits in your safe food routine. Stick with it every time you are out and need to eat. Leave nothing to chance.

FITNESS ROUTINE

The last few chapters of the book are dedicated to this topic. It will become part of your safe zone soon enough if it is not already. To really LIVE in your safe zone, exercise and activity are essential. If you are not in a routine yet, I suggest that you set aside 10 continuous minutes per day at least 5 times per week to do something: walk around the block, walk the stairs at work, dance, bike, treadmill — whatever. This is not about sweat-and-get-short-of-breath exercise yet. This is carving out the space and rhythm of routine for real exercise in the future.

REWARDS PROGRAM

Go back to the chapter on cognitive control. If you have not established your own rewards program yet, now is the time. Review your ideas from that chapter...how can you put these into play?

_____

_____

_____

_____

The beauty of the safe zone is this: when you step outside of your routine, it is obvious to you, and you have a regimen to step back into. The only failure in self-management of adiposity is the failure to step back into your safe zone. As soon as you step back in, the sense of failure stops and self-management is back.

Safe zone is a defined way of living. Maybe boring, sometimes annoying, often frustrating but ALWAYS safe. You may even surprise yourself by how much you really like your safe zone.

CHAPTER 11

INFRASTRUCTURE: EATING OUT

In this chapter you will learn 5 principles for staying within your "safe zone" and making good choices while eating out, where peer-pressure, advertising pressure and sensory stimulation are at their maximum.

ANTICIPATE

Anticipation is about visualizing what the circumstances will be like: what foods may be on offer; how the food will be set up (buffet, self-serve at a table, standing up being offered trays of food/drink, ordering from a menu); if will there be alcohol or other drinks; who will be present and how might they view your food/drink choices. Once you have tried to imagine all of these circumstances, begin building your plan. Plan ahead HOW you will behave and make choices under these circumstances. Make very specific plans such as: *"I know I will be ordering off the menu, so I will only look at the appetizers and choose a small item from there. I will choose one alcoholic drink and ask for it only when the food arrives, and I will say no to breads and desserts right up front by verbalizing this wish to my friends/family/the waitress (whomever is handy!)."*

Think about your next dinner out and do some visualizing and planning:

Where: _____

What foods: _____

_____

Set up: _____

_____

Drinks: _____

The company: _____

_____

MY PLAN: _____

_____

_____

_____

_____

_____

Anticipation is also about choosing your FEELINGS about your food/drink choices... you did not misread that! Sticking with good choices made ahead of time (the "plan") is highly dependent upon your feelings in the situation. Choose the feelings you want to have both going into the circumstance as well as the feelings you wish to have upon leaving. Here is an example: I am writing this chapter from a nice little coffee shop in

Vancouver. Before coming here I had made the plan that I would have coffee and a 100 calorie snack. I chose to feel powerful and in control of my own choices before coming in. I chose to feel happy upon leaving knowing I had kept to my plan (the sequence of face smile, chest smile, and abdomen smile!). Then I saw all these great baked goods and ordered a 400 calorie scone — bad move. But the desire to feel powerful and in control took over before it was too late, so I ripped off ¾ of it and put it in the garbage using my chosen feelings to stick with the plan. I had to do it immediately, though! For those of you who think this is wasteful — you are right. But it is better in the garbage than stored as excess fat tissues that harm the body. It was making a good choice after a bad one before it was too late.

PLAN AHEAD

Do your research before you leave home. Think about what meal you will need to eat while you're out. Go to the web and figure out what food facilities (fast food place, restaurant, cafeteria, et cetera) are available and look over their menus. Use your food logging program to help you figure out the amounts of calories, fats and proteins in the menu items. Then choose the item(s) that meet your needs and allow you to stay in your safe zone. Many people find it helpful to "pre-log" their choices.

Planning for outings: I find it very helpful to have a "go to" fast food place that is widely available so that no matter where I go, I can get a 300 calorie low fat turkey sub with no cheese. This takes care of the danger of eating on the run with minimal planning ahead. Alternatively, I often pack my own lunch so that I get in my 5/5: 8/8, which is otherwise exceedingly difficult to do on the run. "Eat what you pack; pack what you eat."

Try the following exercise to find a "go to" place/food when you are on the run:

Where do I usually find myself when I need a quick meal on the road? (i.e.: burger place, coffee shop, et cetera)

_____

_____

What are the menu choices there that fit within my safe zone?

_____

_____

_____

_____

What alternate food places could I consider?

What foods choices there keep me in my safe zone?

_____

_____

_____

Planning ahead for dining out rather than eating "on the run" requires similar steps. Look up the restaurant menu on the web and figure out what foods you can order that are within your safe zone. Call the restaurant and PRE-order your meal. Making a good food choice in the "moment," even with your work on "anticipation" above, is very difficult. Once the menu is in your hands and the food descriptions seduce you, it is too late to make safe choices. Remember the analogy of the raging river — it's easier to <u>stay</u> out of it than to get out once you are swept up. There are many hidden pressures in dining with friends or family, not the least of which is our very human tendency to imitate others and our desire to fit in. You will not bow to these pressures if you pre-order whenever possible.

Planning ahead for eating at someone's home can be a bit tricky. None of us wish to insult the cook! This is one situation where an email ahead of time is essential. Contact the host; let them know you are on a health plan and that leaving food on your plate and not eating breads or desserts at their event is in no way meant to be hurtful but that these actions are part of your health treatment. You do have a disease. It does have to be managed, all day every day — whether in your own home, someone else's home, the work place or on the go.

BE "THE ONE WHO"

Eating out almost always involves friends or family. Make it your goal to become known as "the one who" only orders salads, does not eat the breads, only has one drink, makes one trip to the buffet etc — you get the idea. This is about intentionally building your identity and reputation as it relates to food choices. For the first few years your friends or family will make comments (positive or negative), but over time your behaviors will be nothing new or different to them — you are just "the one who." Living out this identity in every social eating circumstance will keep you in your safe zone. Maintaining your reputation is a form of self-imposed accountability. More on this in chapter 13.

When I go out to eat, I am the one who_____

_____

_____

_____

REMAIN VIGILANT

Making good decisions around food tends to break down in stages rather than all at once. The first stage of breakdown is due to environmental cues (where visualizing ahead can be exceedingly helpful). The second stage is mindless behavior, and the third stage is a mild form of catastrophizing.

This first stage in breakdown is based on environmental cues. These are the triggers in the dining environment that give our brain a message about food behaviors. For instance, you spent time figuring out your smell triggers in an earlier chapter. Go back to reflect on your homework there. When I smell freshly baked bread, that smell triggers (or cues) my brain to eat in an attempt to recreate feelings of warmth and security in grandma's kitchen. There are all kinds of cues in the dining environment that can lead to a breakdown in decision making — everything from the music, the lighting, the smells and the menu descriptions. Plan in advance how you will manage those triggers by choosing what self-talk will you use. Go back to the self-talk chapter if you need some reminders.

_____

_____

_____

_____

The second stage is mindless behavior. When the cues are working on you, your guard goes down. With your guard let down it is very easy to mindlessly have a couple of someone else's fries, or to have breads or butter, or to let the waiter pour a second alcoholic drink until you find yourself making more and more poor choices. Poor choice behavior that begins mindlessly gradually becomes easier and easier as barriers fall. Once enough barriers to poor decision making fall, poor choices start to become intentional — no longer mindless. This leads to stage 3 – catastrophizing and thereby persisting in intentional poor choices.

Vigilance against mindless behaviors requires careful observation of your "usual" behaviors. Think about past experiences of eating out. What are some of your usual poor choices or behaviors? Make a list of these behaviors and then list ways you can avoid mindlessly engaging in them. Here are some of my examples to get you started:

Mindless Behavior	How to Avoid it
Taking bites of other people's dessert	*Get rid of all utensils after main course*
Eating breads	*Get rid of bread plate upon sitting down*

DR. LORI TEEPLE

The final stage of a "breakdown" in good decision making is catastrophizing. Part of remaining vigilant is to recognize this attitude in yourself and shut it down. If your choices when eating out have been outside your safe zone and have gone from mindless to intentional, you are at a high risk of catastrophizing and carrying on with conscious, ongoing and intentional poor decision making. How can you shut that down and get back on the self-management track? Go back to chapter 8 and the section on catastrophizing — review your ideas. Do it now.

One additional method of shutting down catastrophizing is to do something intentionally positive and active in self-management: Exercise vigorously, purge your kitchen, make a low calorie soup, log as honestly and completely as you can, reset your reward system, or sign a self-management contract with yourself or a friend. Circle what might work for you — it might have to be all of the above.

Vigilance is particularly important under conditions of fatigue, after a glass of wine or when emotions are running strong (anger, sadness, fear, frustration). Recognizing these as added pressures when planning ahead is even more critical.

Reflect

The next 3 or 4 times that you eat out it, is very important afterwards to reflect upon what went well and why and how you felt about it at the time. Write that out — read it every time you go out to reinforce good choices and build upon your repertoire of strategies.

What went well?

Example: I ordered salad _____

_____

_____

_____

Why?

I ordered first and did not listen to what others were ordering _____

_____

_____

_____

How did I feel?

Happy and not deprived _____

_____

_____

_____

Next time eating out: What went well?

_____

_____

_____

_____

Why?

_____

_____

_____

_____

How did I feel?

_____

_____

_____

_____

Next time eating out: What went well?

_____

_____

_____

_____

Why?

_____

_____

_____

_____

How did I feel?

_____

_____

_____

_____

CHAPTER 12

INFRASTRUCTURE: TWINS AND THE EVIL TWIN

Much of our food-related behavior is rooted in habits, associations and circumstances. Over the years I have found that there are 3 main sets of "twins" where food and drink habits are concerned. These are different for everyone. In this chapter you will figure out your "twins" and begin to think of ways to get rid of the so-called "evil" one in each pair.

- Food & Food/Drink & Food Twins

- Activity & Food Twins

- Location & Food Twins

FOOD & FOOD

Think of foods that are within your regimen of self-management, and then think of foods that go along with these that may not be within your safe zone.

Here are some of my examples:

Turkey — Stuffing
Potatoes — Butter/margarine
Strawberries — Shortcake
Salad — Bacon (pancetta) bits

Start building your list of foods that have an "evil twin"
(leave the third column blank for now)

FOOD	EVIL TWIN	CHOICE

Now, in the third column write in substitutes, or decide to drop the evil twin **or** the pair of twins outright.

Here is a sample from my list:

> *Turkey — Stuffing — drop the evil twin*
>
> *Potatoes (rare treat) — Butter/margarine — substitute: lemon juice*
>
> *Strawberry Shortcake — drop the cake evil twin — use lower fat vanilla yogurt*
>
> *Salad — Bacon (pancetta) bits — substitute: shallots chopped up in oil and vinegar*

Here are some examples to get you started on your own list:

Coffee — Cookie/pastry/muffin (the list goes on) — substitute: tbsp. pumpkin seeds on yogurt or 6 almonds

Wine — Cheese and crackers — substitute: olives

Coffee — Cream &/or sugar — make a gradual reduction in amounts — change to milk, drop sugar

Diet Coke — Chips — substitute: tonic water — no food required, or DROP the pair

DRINK	EVIL TWIN	CHOICE

There are some classic examples here:

> *Baseball game — Hot dogs*
>
> *Reception — Wine and cheese*
>
> *Superbowl party — Pizza/chili/chips/beer*
>
> *Campfire — Marshmallows*
>
> *TV or Movie — Popcorn/chips/sodas*

Now it's your turn to reflect on foods/drinks that twin with common activities in your life: (leave the third column blank for now)

ACTIVITY	EVIL TWIN	CHOICE

Carefully consider each set of twins…what skill will you choose to employ? Fill in the initials for each one using the short forms for those skills below:

- Continue the food/drink twin using portion control and skill power (PC-SP)

- Substitute for the food/drink twin (Sub)

- Drop the food/drink twin altogether but keep the activity (Cold Turkey)

- Modify the activity to avoid the food/drink twin (go late, leave early, change time of day) (MOD)

- Stop the activity (STOP)

LOCATION & FOOD

Below is a list of locations that are highly likely to have some "evil" twin food/drink habit attached. Fill in the blanks for the ones that apply to you:

Coffee shop _____

_____

Gas station _____

_____

Your car _____

_____

Lunch room at work _____

_____

Your desk _____

_____

Your favorite chair _____

_____

Grocery store line up _____

_____

Convenience store _____

_____

Pool hall _____

_____

Hockey arena _____

_____

Bar _____

_____

Church _____

_____

Community club _____

_____

Bowling alley _____

_____

List below any additional specific locations with their associated "evil" twin food/drink

_____

_____

_____

_____

_____

_____

_____

_____

_____

_____

_____

_____

Carefully consider each set of twins. What skill will you choose to employ? Fill in the initials for each one using the short forms for those skills below:

- Continue the food/drink twin using portion control and skill power (PC-SP)

- Substitute for the food/drink twin (Sub)

- Drop the food/drink twin altogether but keep the location (Cold Turkey)

- Modify the location to avoid the food/drink twin (buy gas at the pump, detoxify your desk, make a different lunch "room" setting at work) (MOD)

- Avoid the location altogether (STOP)

Spend some time on this chapter, and go back to it each time you identify another "twin scenario" in your own life. This kind of identification allows you full awareness of when, how and how much you might be eating or drinking in a mindless way. Once identified, you have a choice around what to do with the so-called "evil twin." You will need to come back to this chapter and review/revise your lists frequently for the first entire year of self-management. Go through all the seasons and the foods/locations/activities that go with each time of year.

CHAPTER 13

INFRASTRUCTURE: TRAVEL/VACATIONS & CELEBRATIONS

Save this chapter until the week before your next trip/event!

I start writing this chapter from a vacation place — one of those "all-inclusive" places. It is instructive to observe food and drink behaviors, both my own and that of others under conditions of high food/drink availability and variety — particularly at the buffets. What is clear to me is that when there are very few barriers to indulgence, people overindulge — and it's not on broccoli. Here we are in a place of paradise with endless amounts of time to do, well, anything we like…but out of 1000's of guests there are rarely more than 2 or 3 in the gym at a time, and very few out walking/running/playing tennis/et cetera. What's wrong with this picture? Our standard reason for not exercising is lack of time. Our standard reason for eating outside of safe zone is the time required for planning and preparing paired with unpredictable events in our work/home/social life. In this holiday place none of these conditions apply and yet overindulgence and sedentariness are the norm.

What are your thoughts about why this is?

_____

_____

_____

I suspect that there are many powerful influencing factors at play. It is of critical importance to learn to maintain the "safe zone" during vacations, family holiday gatherings and when travelling. The most important reason to maintain the safe zone is this: These are very common conditions under which people revert back to their old way of living and stay there with those old habits rather than continuing with self-management, even if the event is only a weekend long. Understanding and learning to outsmart some of these powerful influencing factors is at the heart of this chapter.

OVERCOMING SOCIAL EXPECTATIONS/NORMS

For almost everyone around us during holidays or celebrations, it's about the food. We speak our love with food. We embrace one another with a drink together. We are accepted into the circle of relationship by "breaking bread" together. We participate in vacation excitement and fun through the shared experience of eating and drinking. None of us wants to stand out as different or be rejected for our "controlled" participation or offend the host or hurt the feelings of others who overindulge and expect the same from us. Those of us doing lifelong self-management are not going to change others. We can change ourselves — our ways of thinking and feeling and doing in these circumstances.

BECOME "THE ONE WHO"

On vacation or travelling or celebrating, how would those who know you well describe you with reference to both foods and activity? Would they say, "He's the one who goes for a jog every day" or "She's the one who drinks only one glass of wine" or "She's the one who uses the small plate for dinner?" It really does not matter what other people think of you. It matters profoundly that you reshape how you see yourself. Do the following exercise as a way to begin thinking of yourself differently and planning the behaviors that support your new identity with respect to eating and exercise. Imagine each circumstance in which you will find yourself during vacation/travel/celebration and plan your choices ahead of time.

Currently I am "the one who"

Example: Samples all the foods on offer _____

_____

_____

Next time I am "the one who"

Example: Chooses a plateful of freggies and just a morsel of one protein/meat/cheese/etc. ____

_____

_____

GETTING CAUGHT UP IN THE MOOD

"It's not about the food." Vacation/travel and celebrations are times when the "mood" heavily influences choices usually dictating excessive eat and drink behaviors as a means of expressing fun and enjoyment. You won't want to change that mood. What you can change is your perspective on what gives you fun and enjoyment. Find other things that give you pleasure. Reframe your ideas about what gives you a sense of fun apart from food and drink. Make a list of things in the travel/vacation/celebration environment that might give you enjoyment. Do this before you are in the midst of the "mood" and risk getting caught up with the poor choices of others. This will help you shift the center of your enjoyment away from the food. Here are some examples. Circle what might be pleasurable for you and then build your own list:

Vacation/travel	Family Celebrations
Moonlight walk	Conversations
Massage	Going for a walk together
Dancing	Playing a board game
Hot tub	Doing a simple craft
Movies	A great book

_____

_____

_____

_____

_____

ACCESS TO GOOD FOOD AND FITNESS

Often when travelling, the availability of foods from the "safe zone" is limited. This has a tremendous influence on choices. Here are my travel tips learned over many years of going on medical courses where the food is almost always low-quality carbohydrates and fats (a source of ironic humor to me is the sugar coated croissants offered for breakfast at a recent diabetes course).

- Always get a hotel room with a mini fridge.

- Find a grocery store near your lodging — load up on freggies, low fat yogurt and cheese.

- Have breakfast from your own groceries in your room.

- Pack your lunch and snacks from your own groceries.

- Do not order room service and eat in front of the TV.

- If the hotel does not have a gym or pool and it is unsafe to jog or walk outside OR you cannot pack your running shoes, bring an exercise DVD or app with you to do in your room when you travel. Even a 10 minute workout will keep you in the rhythm of your "safe zone."

BREAKING NEW GROUND FOR THE SELF

It takes a great deal of effort to change vacation/travel/celebration habits. One powerful negative influence is the tendency to think that these events can be exceptions to your self-management safe zone living. Think again. Think of your next 3 or 4 events as "breaking new ground." Set your expectations and write out very specific plans. Choose a reward that will help you stick to your plans. Choose a mantra — look at the self-talk chapter for ideas.

Expectation:

_____

_____

_____

_____

Plans:

_____

_____

_____

_____

Reward:

_____

_____

_____

_____

Mantra (self-talk):

_____

_____

_____

_____

Finally, one of the most frequent comments I am given by those who have gotten out of safe zone on vacation is this: "I walked a lot so it sort of made up for the extra food." There are numerous studies demonstrating that we almost always overestimate the amount of calories burned in activity — by 3 or 4 times. How far does one need to walk to "burn off" the average burger and fries or steak and Caesar salad? Give it your best guess.

Here is the math: the average burger and fries is about 1000 calories, as is an 8 oz steak with Caesar salad. The average person must walk about 20 km to "burn off" those calories (walking very briskly for 4 hours at 5 km/hr with no breaks). I would have to run for 1.5 hours at about 10 km/hr — or 15 km. Activity and exercise are not about burning calories or losing weight. Exercise and "moving" are extremely important for metabolism, muscle building, bone preservation and overall health — and weight loss will not be kept off without exercise — but activity or outright exercise is not a "make-up" for poor food choices.

RETURNING TO ROUTINES

Don't read this section until you return from travel.

All is not lost if the safe zone is blown on vacation. All is never lost. Start back in the safe zone. Re-read the 7 Essentials, give yourself the first 2 days back and then begin to weigh yourself daily. Logging is the most important device for re-establishing safe zone. Decide right now to go on your logging website and just start again — decide when and where you will do your logging. Set a new goal. Devise a new reward. If you do not feel like exercising because you are out of your routine, just put on your fitness clothes and your runners, go out the door, walk around for a minute, do some self-talk and see what happens. Do it now.

CHECK IN

Very few of us with adiposity can sustain self-management by knowledge alone. The 7 Essentials and skill power are the backbone of creating and maintaining a lifestyle in the "safe zone." Go back to chapter 3 – how are you doing with the 7 Essentials (and weighing daily)? Give yourself a report card right now:

Breakfast _____/100. Anything need to change?
What do you need to do to make it happen?

_____

_____

_____

_____

Logging _____/100. If it is not happening, ask yourself why — then figure out what you need to do to make it happen.

_____

_____

_____

_____

Exercise _____/100. Anything need to change? What do you need to do to make it happen ONE more time per week?

_____

_____

_____

_____

90% of foods eaten at home or packed up from home _____/100. Anything need to change? What do you need to do to make it happen?

_____

_____

_____

_____

Always measure portions _____/100. Is it happening? What needs to change?

_____

_____

_____

_____

5/5: 8/8_____/100. Is it happening? Figure out why not and how can you fix it.

_____

_____

_____

_____

3 meals and 2 or 3 snacks per day_____/100. Is this happening? Figure out a way.

_____

_____

_____

_____

Weigh Daily_____/100. If you don't do this, think about why and journal it here. This is an important question for you right now. Weighing (or measuring the waist) is a daily ritual of commitment designed to keep you out of denial.

_____

_____

_____

_____

CHAPTER 14

MOVEMENT: EXERCISE

There are 3 forms of "movement" in self-management of adiposity. We will cover activity/mobility in the next chapter and moving to a safe zone in the following one.

Earlier in the book, I mentioned the benefits of exercise for the control of adiposity. It is rare for someone to lose weight based solely on exercise. And it is rare for someone to keep off the weight they lose unless they <u>do</u> exercise. Remember those folks on the weight control registry? The successful losers who keep their weight off do daily exercise. Too much muscle mass is lost in the process of losing weight unless "real" exercise (*as defined below*) is routine. Too much bone mass is lost unless exercise is routine. Weight will be regained unless exercise is routine, guaranteed.

The biggest barrier to exercise is not lack of time, lack of money, distance from a gym, sore joints, a bad back or being too heavy to do anything. These are barriers no doubt, but none are insurmountable.

Write out a list of your "barriers" to exercise. Remember that exercise is distinct from activity in 2 major ways:

1. Intensity

2. Duration (10 minutes at a time minimum / total 150 minutes per week)

Intensity refers to "getting sweaty and short of breath." When I discuss a walking program with a patient who has diabetes, I do not mean going for a walk. I mean walking to the intensity of breathing so hard it is difficult to hold a conversation and sweating from the effort. I do not mean walking the dog or walking the golf course. These are great activities but they are not "exercise."

What are your barriers to "real" exercise?

_____

_____

_____

_____

The biggest barrier is motivation. It is hard. Sometimes it is very hard to dredge up the energy, the will, and the drive to exercise. Just as with food choices, will power is not enough. We need skill power. The skills of self-motivation for exercise fall into 3 categories:

1. Reward

2. Twinning

3. Challenging oneself

REWARD

Exercise (getting sweaty and short of breath for 10 minutes at a time — totalling 150 mins per week) is hard work — for some it feels like drudgery, like just one more task to incorporate into an already busy life. Initiating and sustaining any project demands that the reward is continually worth the effort. There are four kinds of rewards as motivation.

IMMEDIATE REWARD

Set up a system for yourself whereby doing the exercise you planned on earns you a "reward" — something immediate, visible, tangible, audible and cumulative. A common suggestion is to put coins or buttons in a glass jar. At our clinic we put magnets on a white board next to our name for every day we exercise. At the end of a week, having accumulated those visible/tangible/audible rewards marking your efforts, add the next level of reward. It is critically important to have an immediate reward system. Do not skip this habit. Your brain is starving for these rewards to feed the process of undergoing changes of habit.

What are some immediate reward ideas that would work for you:

_____

_____

_____

_____

_____

_____

INTERMEDIATE/LONGER TERM REWARD

After a week or a month of immediate reward accumulation it is time for you to collect on your prize. Make that prize something you can truly anticipate with excitement or pleasure for the entire week or month in advance. For some it will be a new golf club or a new pair of shoes. For others it will be a spa treatment or going out to a show. Some people might buy a ten dollar traveller's cheque each week or month and watch the stack of them grow aiming for a vacation. Decide what would be a special reward for you. Then start the whole process over again perhaps with a different "end of week/month" prize.

_____

_____

_____

_____

_____

PREDICTED REWARDS

When I am finding it especially difficult to put on my runners to get out for a jog or go into the garage to lift weights, I will ask myself a motivator question. "What 3 good things will happen if I exercise right now?" The answers might vary with the day but generally will be along the lines of this: 1) I will be really happy with myself when I'm done, 2) I will fit my pants, and 3) If I do this now it will be easier the next time.

How might you answer this question for yourself?
"What 3 good things will happen if I exercise right now?"

_____

_____

_____

_____

_____

ENDORPHIN AND ENERGY REWARDS

It is absolutely true that exercising regularly raises levels of endorphins, the so-called happiness hormones, and energy. On the scale provided, rate your level of energy at mid-afternoon most days. After six weeks of immediate and longer term rewards, come back to the scale and rate your energy level. If it has not improved, bump up the intensity of your work out — add in some resistance training (weights, calisthenics, machines) and ensure you are getting 5/5: 8/8 without eating any cheap carbs. Return to the scale a month later, and I guarantee your energy score will be substantially higher. Your endorphin happy mood should be as well.

$$\longleftrightarrow$$

0	5	10
no energy — feel like sleeping	enough energy to make dinner & do laundry	energy to exercise & do laundry & go to a show

TWINNING

Earlier in the book, you learned that creating a new habit is much easier when you attach it to an old habit. This is one of the ways that our brain retrains itself. Another such mechanism is to attach a new habit to something very positive. For example, when I hear my Bryan Adams CD (positive for me) I totally feel like doing a fitness routine (dance or weights) because I have combined the two for so long; twinning is working for me. Destination twins work well — if I need to motivate myself to go for a long bike ride or run I choose a nice coffee destination, which is a positive twin for me. Time efficiency twins work well — if you are waiting on someone (kids at music lessons or sports events), take 15 minutes and exercise. You will feel positive about your time management. Meeting up with a friend to do exercise can be a positive twin. A new exercise shirt can be a positive twin. There are many "twins" you can set up that will positively attract you to your exercise routine. Reflect on some "positive twins" you can create to attract you to exercise:

_____

_____

_____

_____

_____

_____

Conversely, if your exercise environment is uninspiring or downright discouraging it can act as a negative twin, so — change it. Make a list of what is turning you off and what alternatives you can imagine — I'll get you started:

Currently negative twin	Alternative
I hate exercising in the basement; no daylight	*Move treadmill to garage with window*

CHALLENGING YOURSELF

There is no "best" exercise. The best one for you is the one you will **do**. Start there. Start realistically. If you do not already have an exercise routine then start with 5 minutes per day of an exercise you know you can do. Expect to feel sore — soreness in muscles is good, embrace it before, during and after you exercise. Stretching before, during and after is truly advisable. Warming up is essential at higher levels of intensity. There are all kinds of websites and books to advise you on this. My mission is to help you get motivated and stay motivated. Motivation involves "purpose." While the overall purpose of exercise is self-management of adiposity (aka good health), the day-to-day motivation must have a more tangible purpose. Additionally, the more fit you become the more you will need to exert yourself to "get short of breath and sweaty" ("real" exercise).

DISTANCE CHALLENGE

If you jog, run or walk 1 km now — set yourself up for the challenge of doing 1.5 km in 2 weeks — then 2 km in a month — then 3 km in 2 months. Go as far as you choose. Once you have reached your distance challenge, go for a time or skill challenge. Go now and get a calendar, write the distances you expect to be doing in 1 week, then 2, then 3. Send yourself email reminders or post the schedule on the fridge.

TIME CHALLENGE

If you do your run or bike ride in an hour now, set yourself up for the challenge of doing it in 50 minutes at the end of 4 weeks, then 45 minutes in 8 weeks, et cetera. Once you have reached your time challenge look at a distance challenge or add a skill challenge.

SKILL CHALLENGE

Variety in exercise is really important not just for psychological/motivation reasons but for muscle balance and development, injury prevention, remaining flexible in the back and joints, et cetera. Learning and doing a variety of exercises is the skill challenge. If you have always been a walker, you may choose to try a step class. If you have always done stationary biking, you may choose swimming. You get the idea. Having a variety of exercise routines is paramount to sustaining lifelong self-management. Finding the routines that suit you may take a year of challenging yourself with new exercises. Go for it. Make a list of possible exercises you could try:

_____

_____

_____

_____

_____

_____

One of the essential skill challenges is to learn a resistance exercise regime. Resistance exercise is not so much "get short of breath and sweaty" as in walking, jogging, biking. Resistance exercise is slower, more sustained muscle movement usually against a force. Examples: push-ups, squats, weight lifting, weight machines, et cetera. You do not actually need to join a gym or buy equipment to do resistance training (although lots of people enjoy going to a gym — whatever is a positive twin for you, go for it). You can simply use your own bodyweight as "resistance." A slick routine is 10 moves x 1 minute each in your own home (I like setting the cell phone timer for each minute). Think of all the moves you can do without equipment. Look up good technique or hire a trained fitness instructor for a session to learn proper technique. You could include push-ups, planks, squats, lunges, sit ups, crunches, burpees, tricep dips from a chair, chair rises, et cetera. Make a list — see what works for you. Try out the "7 minute workout" app.

_____

_____

_____

_____

_____

_____

STRENGTH CHALLENGE

Once you have a resistance routine (two to three sessions per week — about 15 to 20 minutes each time), the way to keep it fresh and "motivating" is to add purpose to the routine. If you are doing 10 push-ups now add another 2 for the next 3 workouts, or add another 2 sit ups to the routine, or another 2 lbs to the weights if you use them. Always be building onto the workout — challenge yourself with heavier, or longer, or more repetitions. Make it a little "competition" with yourself.

COMPETITION CHALLENGE

There is nothing quite so motivating as preparing for an event such as a fundraiser 5 km walk/run or a half marathon. Choose an event and work toward just doing it without concern for how you stack up against others. Stop right now, look up on the web what kinds of events are happening in your locale 2 months from now, 4 months from now, and 6 months from now. Choose a few of these, register, and start your "training" all in the name of motivating yourself.

_____

_____

_____

_____

_____

_____

_____

Use all 3 motivators all the time for the rest of your life — rewards, twins and challenging yourself. If all else fails, I generally just put on my running shoes, walk out the door and tell myself just to jog to the end of the laneway. If I do this, just plan to get that far and allow myself the option to quit and walk back by the end of the laneway, I almost always decide to keep on jogging!

CHAPTER 15

MOVEMENT: MOVING OUT OF THE DANGER ZONES

Think for a few minutes right now about all of the locations in which you find yourself eating. From the list below, circle the ones that are a "danger zone" for you. A danger zone is a location where you find yourself eating outside of your planned, safe routine. There will be some overlap here with the chapter on twins. However, this skill is all about "movement."

HOME

Kitchen (standing up at the counter, the fridge or the cupboard — not your usual sit-down eating place)

TV room

Computer/desk

Bed

Other _____

OUT AND ABOUT

Gas station

Variety/corner store

Arena/sports field

Drive-thru fast food

Coffee shop

Food court

Other _____

WORK

Desk

Computer

Lunch room

Cafeteria

Other _____

Start with "home" and start with "kitchen" for the following exercise — this is the kind of exercise that you will need to repeat for all of your danger zones. It might take you a few months to recognize these zones and develop your "exit strategies" for movement away from each one.

Kitchen: break this down into areas of the kitchen — do you open the fridge door and do unplanned eating? Is it the freezer door? Is it a certain cupboard or two? These are the kitchen hotspots usually. Picture yourself in your hotspot. Then picture yourself walking away — plan where you will go and what you will do in a different location in your house. Move away from the kitchen and force yourself to stay in your alternate location when the time comes to enact your plan. It's all about moving away and staying away. And it is about having a "go to" alternative place. You may need to change your location habits. Here is an example — over the last 8 months I have been doing work from home sitting at the kitchen table. I began to realize what a danger zone that is for me when I noticed how often I was at the fridge or the coffee-maker (which generally leads to eating anything I can get my hands on). I have changed to a different work room — it required my finding a lap board on which to work, but the change of "venue" alone has altered the desire to eat outside my safe zone by limiting access and cues.

Where are your danger zones in your house? You can identify these using little sticky notes to mark where you are when you are eating out of safe zone. In order to break the pattern you will need to develop an alternate plan/location. For example, if you find yourself raiding the fridge before bed, look at the other things you do before bed — do you go get into your pajamas? Do you stop in the kitchen on your way from the TV room? Do you go to the sink for water? Do you pack your lunch for the next day? Look at all the activities or patterns that lead up to the eating you do not plan to do. Then find a way to change the pattern and stay out of or get quickly out of the kitchen.

Danger Location 1: _____

Time of day: _____

Patterns leading up to: _____

_____

NEW patterns/alternative locations (exit strategy):_____

_____

Danger Location 2: _____

Time of day: _____

Patterns leading up to: _____

_____

NEW patterns/alternative locations (exit strategy): _____

_____

Danger Location 3: _____

Time of day: _____

Patterns leading up to: _____

_____

NEW patterns/alternative locations (exit strategy): _____

_____

_____

Danger Location 4: _____

Time of day: _____

Patterns leading up to: _____

_____

NEW patterns/alternative locations (exit strategy): _____

_____

SOCIAL EVENTS

Position yourself away from the food. Find a location where you must make a big effort to get food. Think ahead and remind yourself of the importance of strategic location. If the food is mainly on a table in someone's dining room or on a counter at a work event or drinks are on the bar, position yourself in another room or as far away as possible. Draw an invisible circle for yourself from that location and stick within that circle for the whole event. Ask a friend to bring you a drink or a small snack rather than being triggered into mindless eating and poor choices by moving into the danger zone.

JUST KEEP MOVING

There will be times that you do not have an "exit strategy" from a danger zone. In this situation it is best to focus on moving on — just keep moving, whether that is walking or driving. Do not focus on the argument within directing you to indulge in eating which is not in your safe zone. Focus on the movement away from. Consciously reward your behavior with the face smile — chest smile — abdominal smile. Reinforce the behavior for next time.

CHAPTER 16

MOVEMENT: ACTIVITY AND MOBILITY, SEDENTARY NO MORE

Activity is distinct from exercise. We need both. Generally speaking, activity is about moving rather than the sustained "get short of breath and sweaty" of true exercise. There are two ways of looking at activity in order to incorporate more of it into your life — sedentary time and movement time.

SEDENTARY

Look at how much time you spend in a sedentary state, like sitting (or lying) per day (other than to sleep). The Canadian Society for Exercise Physiology guidelines for young adults recommends less than 2 hours per day of screen time (includes computer time, TV, video games etc). If a typical movie is 90 to 120 minutes long you can do the math — that leaves less than 30 minutes more of sedentary screen time for the day! Recent research suggests that prolonged sitting (sometimes called "sitting disease") on its own is a risk factor for cardiovascular disease and other health problems even for those who have an exercise routine. Fortunately, it also suggests that breaking up the sitting time by getting up to move frequently can reduce some of those risks to health. Look at your typical day and reflect on the amount of time you spend sitting.

Eating: _____

Travel: _____

Desk work: _____

Reading: _____

Watching a screen: _____

Other: _____

Now figure out a way to break up the sitting time. For me, sitting at work is broken up by having the fax machine across the hall, having the blood pressure cuff across the room, putting the hand washing solution on a shelf away from my desk — all of these little things force me to move. Remember, this section is just about reducing sitting time. For each of the categories think of at least one way to break up the sitting by standing +/- moving.

Eating: _____

Travel: _____

Desk work: _____

Reading: _____

Watching a screen: _____

Other: _____

Dr. Mike Evans has suggested that Canadians start a movement called "make your day harder" (watch it on YouTube "Let's Make Our Day Harder"). He describes the parking spot farthest from the store as the one that is reserved for those who want to live longer and enjoy better health! Seriously, his video is filled with great ideas for increasing activity in daily routines. This will not happen for you unless you plan it — reflect on where and how you can increase your activity level by breaking down your typical schedule.

Getting up in the morning and out the door:

eg: *stretch while the coffee brews*

_____

_____

_____

_____

Transportation to work/school/store:

_____

_____

_____

_____

Lunch hour:

_____

_____

_____

_____

Transportation/travel home:

_____

_____

_____

_____

House or yard work (less automation, more muscle)

_____

_____

_____

_____

FITBIT: I have recently begun using a little monitor called "fitbit" that I wear either as a watch or an ankle bracelet. It tracks my steps per day (and connected online has a good food tracker for logging) and whether those steps are vigorous enough to qualify as exercise. It has been highly motivating and educational. I think I am a very active person — some days when I first began to wear the bracelet my daily steps were nowhere near 10,000, which is a standard recommendation for adult activity. Unless I intentionally plan to take steps they do not happen. This gizmo is worth every penny. You can find it online at www.fitbit.com

FUN AND SOCIALIZING THROUGH ACTIVITY

About 15 years ago some friends invited me to go cycling with them. All I had for a bike was an old mountain bike with cobwebs between the spokes. I dug it out and joined them on a 10 km trek. I was very proud of myself. I never imagined being able to go so far. I never imagined how much I would enjoy chatting and sharing the experience with friends. Cycling has since become not only one of my key social activities, but it has become the main way I do vacations and see the country. Doing holiday time and free time <u>actively</u> is a paradigm shift. When you plan your next trip, start with what activity you want to do — then plan for the destination. Make your vacation or free time about play — physical, active play. Find active things you like to do with friends or family and capitalize on it. They could be things you have done in the past, activities that your friends or family members enjoy, or activities you are interested in trying for fun.

Use this exercise to help you think about your next step:

What activity CAN I do: _____

What did I enjoy doing in the past: _____

What do my friends do (or what can I talk them into doing) : _____

_____

_____

_____

What one activity can I learn to do this year: _____

What activity can I see myself doing for vacation: _____

CHAPTER 17

EMOTIONAL EATING AND ADDICTIVE BEHAVIOUR

I am indebted in this final chapter to Dr. Gabor Maté. He is a Canadian physician who has worked and written extensively about addiction. I will quote frequently from his book *In the Realm of Hungry Ghosts*. This book helped me understand how much of my adiposity is about addiction and Dr. Maté caused me to ask myself some very hard, but important, questions. I still ask them of myself. This chapter is your chance to ask yourself some hard questions. It is my hope that it will help you start figuring out the reasons you sometimes eat out of control. This is just a start. If you are having difficulty, it may just be time to see a trained therapist — seriously, your disease is that important.

You may not be an "emotional" eater; you may not have addictive behavior. You can decide once you have done some of these exercises. This chapter, or rather your reflections, can become a resource for you to review over the year to come. When you find yourself living outside your safe zone and feeling unmotivated or when you find it impossible to get on track in spite of using all the techniques and strategies you have learned, it might just be time to explore or re-explore is going on in your heart and mind.

Dr. Maté says, "Any passion can become an addiction; but then how to distinguish between the two? The central question is: who's in charge, the individual or their behaviour? It's possible to rule a passion, but an obsessive passion that a person is unable to rule is an addiction. And the addiction is the repeated behaviour that a person keeps engaging in, even though he knows it harms himself or others"(pg. 109). Think about this question for yourself in light of some of your eating behaviors (what I call aberrant, out-of-control eating or eating outside your safe zone). In what ways is this description true for you?

_____

_____

_____

_____

_____

_____

_____

_____

_____

_____

_____

Eating out of "need" is not a quest for pleasure (food as pleasure is not addiction) — using food as a "substance" is an attempt to escape from distress. How do you know that you are using food as a "substance?" Think about the last time you were putting something in your mouth and felt like you could not stop although you wanted to stop and you knew intellectually that you should stop. When this happens next time ask yourself, "What is the distress I am attempting to escape?" Your answer may vary depending on your circumstances — leave room for further reflection in the future.

_____

_____

_____

_____

_____

_____

_____

_____

_____

_____

_____

_____

_____

What do you really think food will do for you? Food is meant to nourish your body and provide the pleasure of taste and fellowship with others. When you use food for any other reason — particularly when it is out of control — ask yourself this: *Food, this food at this time in this amount makes a promise to me that it cannot deliver.* What is the false promise it makes?

_____

_____

_____

_____

_____

_____

_____

"Dismissing addictions as 'bad habits' or 'self-destructive behaviour,' comfortably hides their functionality in the life of the addict" (Vincent Felitti, MD, pg. 33). Eating out-of-control has a function in your life — do not dismiss it as just 'bad habits.' Think about the <u>function</u> of so-called addictive eating in your life:

_____

_____

_____

_____

_____

_____

_____

_____

"Hurt is at the center of all addictive behavior" (pg. 36). How does this quote strike you? In what ways does it describe you?

_____

_____

_____

_____

_____

_____

_____

_____

_____

_____

"It's hard to get enough of something that almost works." (Felitti, pg. 101). Let me give you a recent example: I worked a 10 hour day at the clinic, got in the car to drive to my monthly education night in the city, drove about 10 km out of town and was called

back to do a house call for someone who was very sick. This resulted not only in the house call but two trips to the clinic to get equipment and supplies. By the time I got home (and did not get to education night), it was 9 pm. Three bowls of ice cream later (and I don't even like ice cream), I was still feeling self-pity and frustration. Not quite as much as I was before bowl one or two or three — so would another bowl do the trick? The problem with food as consolation is that it "almost" works, so if a little bit helps, maybe even more will help even more. But it is never enough nor can it be. Feeding an emotional need with physical food is like taking antibiotics for a sprained ankle. Wrong treatment. In fact, it makes things worse.

What foods "almost work" for you?

_____

_____

_____

Emotional eating is a food addiction. Emotions that are distressing need to be relieved somehow. Certain foods actually cause a spike in brain "happy" chemicals (like dopamine) and relieve distress — so the food behavior is repeated over and over when distressing emotions arise in spite of the negative consequences of all this eating. Do you ever wonder why the foods eaten in an out-of-control manner are either high in fat or sugar, rather than foods like broccoli or canned tomatoes? Some foods really do produce a little "high" — a boost in emotional energy.

Think about the "distress" you are trying to escape using food or the "high" that you need and then imagine alternative means that actually work (meditation for example) — you may need a skilled counsellor to help you with this:

_____

_____

_____

_____

_____

_____

_____

_____

If you are spending emotional energy and getting nothing in return, you will end up trying to recoup that loss by ingesting calories unless you figure out some alternatives.

"In the addicted mode, the emotional charge is in the pursuit and the acquisition of the desired object (food) not in…the enjoyment of it." (pg. 107)

How true is this for you? Think back to the last time you ate in an addictive mode. Did you enjoy it? Was the "lift" it gave you about enjoyment? Why not?

_____

_____

_____

_____

_____

_____

_____

_____

"Two things alcoholics hate is work and time. There has to be no effort involved, and you want the results right now." (pg 119)

In what ways have you observed yourself like this regarding self-management of adiposity?

_____

_____

_____

_____

_____

_____

_____

_____

"The distinguishing features of any addiction are: compulsion, preoccupation, impaired control, persistence, relapse and craving" *(Pg 214).*

Let me narrate a scenario to illustrate these elements — then you will have a turn to analyze your own food addiction behavior using these 6 features.

This is one of my own recurring scenarios: Late in the evening, after an event in the city, I have a long drive home. I have this overwhelming urge to stop for chips and Diet Coke. I talk myself down, I pass a few corner stores and gas stations, but I am so preoccupied with getting chips that I cannot think of anything else (if you don't have food addiction you are probably thinking "this woman is a bit nuts"). I finally stop at a gas station. I buy the chips — sometimes 2 bags. I eat them in the car, alone, then ashamed. I hide the bag(s) under the seat. I persist in this behavior many times when I am driving alone at night. But I really try to avoid it — to have alternatives in the car, to plan a driving route that does not have gas stations or corner stores. I do really well for a month or so, then I relapse. The craving is just too great — the compulsion sets in again....

Think about one of your own repetitive aberrant food behaviors. Write out the scenario and observe for the 6 elements (compulsion, preoccupation, impaired control, persistence, relapse and craving).

_____

_____

_____

_____

_____

_____

_____

_____

_____

_____

_____

_____

_____

Now, go back and circle two steps in your scenario where you could "interrupt" the circuit. For example, in my own scenario I could interrupt the behavior at the point of planning my driving route, I could interrupt it by phoning home and talking (hands free) en route until all the dangerous gas stations are behind me…you get the idea. Figure out possible interruptions to your cycle of behavior. If you have more than one of these scenarios in your repertoire, do the same exercise for each one. It is worth your time. Do it now. Beyond figuring out in the previous exercises the "whys" of addictive eating behaviours, this exercise is meant to add some practical steps and strategies. What "interruptions" are you planning in your scenario?

_____

_____

_____

_____

_____

_____

_____

_____

_____

_____

_____

Do you recall being in high school and unable to do a certain subject (let's say math or typing)? Can you recall saying in exasperation and defeat "I just can't do it?" What was the objective in that? Was it to get you off the hook? Was it about finding a reason not to do the hard work? Was it about excusing yourself from the time and effort (and frustration)? Those were my objectives in saying "I just can't do it" regarding grade 11 math. That was a lie I told myself. Truth is, a few years later when I wanted to get into medical school I could do math like a whiz. What changed? I did not suddenly get smarter. My motivation changed. Truth is, the ability was there all along.

It really is time to tell yourself the truth about being able to do self-management of your adiposity and about being able to overcome some of your own addictive behaviors.

This last exercise is intended to help you recognize truth from lies in your own life. Here you are going to make two lists. One is to help you capture the lies you tell yourself. The other is to help you analyse those lies so you can capture the truth. You will need to review the truth column over and over again for the foreseeable future like every time you are tempted to say, "I just can't do it."

Lies I Tell Myself	The Truth
e.g. 1: *My adiposity doesn't really matter.*	e.g. 1: *It is slowly killing me and ruining my health and future.*
e.g. 2: *It's okay to overeat this one time.*	eg 2: *A one-time lapse matters and it matters now.*

Lies are about denial of the reality we do not wish to face.

"Truth will set you free."

RECAP • REVIEW • REFLECT

In Chapter 3 you asked yourself: Why do I want to get to a healthier weight? Before you go back to check your answer there, write down your answer to it here:

_____

_____

_____

_____

_____

Now go back and check Chapter 3...what has changed in your outlook? What has changed in your motivation:

_____

_____

_____

_____

_____

Which of the 7 essentials are going well for you now? Check off the ones that are just a normal part of your life — your safe zone. Circle the ones where you are still struggling.

Breakfast

Logging

Exercise

Eat at home or food packed at home 90% of the time

Measure portions

5/5: 8/8

3 meals and 2 to 3 snacks per day

....and weighing daily (this is just an "odometer" — a ritual reminding you that weight management is one of your important conscious daily priorities).

You will recall from chapter 3 that the successful weight losers/managers on the National Weight Control Registry have proven that these are the habits that lead to life-long weight control. If you and I are going to self-manage this disease, these must be our habits as well.

Reflect on the elements above that you circled...think of these as your next project. Choose one and focus on it. Go back through your book and look again at strategies that you can employ. There is no such thing as failure in self-management of adiposity — the most important skill is just to start over again and use what you learned from getting off track to inform new strategies and avoid pitfalls in the future.

APPENDIX 1

Body Mass Index Table

	Normal						Overweight					Obese										Extreme Obesity														
BMI	19	20	21	22	23	24	25	26	27	28	29	30	31	32	33	34	35	36	37	38	39	40	41	42	43	44	45	46	47	48	49	50	51	52	53	54
Height (inches)												Body Weight (pounds)																								
58	91	96	100	105	110	115	119	124	129	134	138	143	148	153	158	162	167	172	177	181	186	191	196	201	205	210	215	220	224	229	234	239	244	248	253	258
59	94	99	104	109	114	119	124	128	133	138	143	148	153	158	163	168	173	178	183	188	193	198	203	208	212	217	222	227	232	237	242	247	252	257	262	267
60	97	102	107	112	118	123	128	133	138	143	148	153	158	163	168	174	179	184	189	194	199	204	209	215	220	225	230	235	240	245	250	255	261	266	271	276
61	100	106	111	116	122	127	132	137	143	148	153	158	164	169	174	180	185	190	195	201	206	211	217	222	227	232	238	243	248	254	259	264	269	275	280	285
62	104	109	115	120	126	131	136	142	147	153	158	164	169	175	180	186	191	196	202	207	213	218	224	229	235	240	246	251	256	262	267	273	278	284	289	295
63	107	113	118	124	130	135	141	146	152	158	163	169	175	180	186	191	197	203	208	214	220	225	231	237	242	248	254	259	265	270	278	282	287	293	299	304
64	110	116	122	128	134	140	145	151	157	163	169	174	180	186	192	197	204	209	215	221	227	232	238	244	250	256	262	267	273	279	285	291	296	302	308	314
65	114	120	126	132	138	144	150	156	162	168	174	180	186	192	198	204	210	216	222	228	234	240	246	252	258	264	270	276	282	288	294	300	306	312	318	324
66	118	124	130	136	142	148	155	161	167	173	179	186	192	198	204	210	216	223	229	235	241	247	253	260	266	272	278	284	291	297	303	309	315	322	328	334
67	121	127	134	140	146	153	159	166	172	178	185	191	198	204	211	217	223	230	236	242	249	255	261	268	274	280	287	293	299	306	312	319	325	331	338	344
68	125	131	138	144	151	158	164	171	177	184	190	197	203	210	216	223	230	236	243	249	256	262	269	276	282	289	295	302	308	315	322	328	335	341	348	354
69	128	135	142	149	155	162	169	176	182	189	196	203	209	216	223	230	236	243	250	257	263	270	277	284	291	297	304	311	318	324	331	338	345	351	358	365
70	132	139	146	153	160	167	174	181	188	195	202	209	216	222	229	236	243	250	257	264	271	278	285	292	299	306	313	320	327	334	341	348	355	362	369	376
71	136	143	150	157	165	172	179	186	193	200	208	215	222	229	236	243	250	257	265	272	279	286	293	301	308	315	322	329	338	343	351	358	365	372	379	386
72	140	147	154	162	169	177	184	191	199	206	213	221	228	235	242	250	258	265	272	279	287	294	302	309	316	324	331	338	346	353	361	368	375	383	390	397
73	144	151	159	166	174	182	189	197	204	212	219	227	235	242	250	257	265	272	280	288	295	302	310	318	325	333	340	348	355	363	371	378	386	393	401	408
74	148	155	163	171	179	186	194	202	210	218	225	233	241	249	256	264	272	280	287	295	303	311	319	326	334	342	350	358	365	373	381	389	396	404	412	420
75	152	160	168	176	184	192	200	208	216	224	232	240	248	256	264	272	279	287	295	303	311	319	327	335	343	351	359	367	375	383	391	399	407	415	423	431
76	156	164	172	180	189	197	205	213	221	230	238	246	254	263	271	279	287	295	304	312	320	328	336	344	353	361	369	377	385	394	402	410	418	426	435	443

Source: Adapted from *Clinical Guidelines on the Identification, Evaluation, and Treatment of Overweight and Obesity in Adults: The Evidence Report.*

DR. LORI TEEPLE

———————

Dr. Lori Teeple is an associate professor of Medicine and Family Medicine at Western University where she is an award winning teacher. She has been a family and emergency medicine physician for over 25 years and lectures nationally and internationally. Her passion for preventive medicine through healthy lifestyle arises from this work and from her own long term battle with "The disease of overweight"

Printed in Canada